Reconstructive Lymph Vascular Surgery

Ruediger G.H. Baumeister

Reconstructive Lymph Vascular Surgery

Springer

Ruediger G.H. Baumeister
Division of Plastic-, Hand-, and Microsurgery
Department of Surgery
Ludwig Maximilians University
Munich
Germany

ISBN 978-3-319-31645-1 ISBN 978-3-319-31647-5 (eBook)
DOI 10.1007/978-3-319-31647-5

Library of Congress Control Number: 2016941934

Printed on acid-free paper

This Springer imprint is published by Springer Nature
The registered company is Springer International Publishing AG Switzerland

To my family

Preface

The lymphatic vascular system is rarely considered as a field of vascular surgery. Treatment of arteries and veins in open procedures are mostly performed with naked eyes.

However, only with the help of operating microscopes and advanced microsurgical skills that it is possible to deal with lymphatic vessels, like dealing with other vessels in order to perform lymphatic anastomoses and lymphatic bypass procedures.

The necessity to overcome local interruptions of a lymphatic pathway is clinically obvious when lymphedema is the result. Such a lymphatic obstacle may be the sequela of a trauma or a medical intervention, preferentially at regions where the lymphatic transporting system becomes narrow like in the axilla or in the groin area.

Treatment of lymphedema is one of the topics in plastic surgery. There, using the operating microscope to deal with small arteries and veins is a prerequisite for many modern procedures.

Thus, the author, who has a degree in vascular surgery and in plastic surgery as well, was influenced by both disciplines, in the search for a causal therapy for lymphedema caused by a local obstruction of the lymphatic system.

Lymphatic vascular surgery is not restricted to the treatment lymphedema due to local obstacles; it is also important in the reconstruction of damaged lymphatic vessels which may result to lymphoceles or lymph fistulas.

The book gives an overview of the field of reconstructive vascular surgery, performed in our institution, from bench to bedside.

It reflects the pathophysiologic basis of this kind of treatment, shows the experimental basis, and gives hints for training of lymphatic vascular microsurgery. It delivers the ways of investigating the effects of the treatment and shows the results of treatment in patients. Finally, it reflects possible interactions between lymphatic vascular surgery and other treatment options.

The book is primarily addressed to vascular surgeons, plastic surgeons, and interested lymphologists.

It might be helpful to perform lymphatic vascular surgery and to get informed about the possibilities of treating patients by that way.

Munich, Germany — Ruediger G.H. Baumeister

Acknowledgments

Working for the development of a new strategy is never a one-man show. There are supporters who help one to get started, helpers working to establish and colleagues helping to carry on.

The first glimpse to the abdominal thoracic duct of a rat was contrived to me by Prof. Sun Lee from San Diego. At the very end of a microsurgical course in Berlin late at night, he asked: "Who is interested to deal with lymphatic vessels?" Only a few where.

Back in Munich, starting with lymph vascular microsurgery was essentially supported by the head of the Institute for Surgical Research, Prof. Walter Brendel. He was interested in the lymphatic system and had invented the "antilymphocytic serum" to minimize rejection in organ transplantation, a serum which was asked for by Prof. Barnard to treat his heart transplantation patients. In this institute, with the help of a grant, given by the VW foundation, experimental studies were carried out for several years. Valuable help was provided by Prof. J. Seifert from the Institute for Surgical Research, Prof. B. Wiebecke from the Institute of Pathology, and Prof. H. Liebich from the Veterinary Faculty.

One person has to be mentioned specifically in this context: Mrs. Jutta Krumbach, a chemotechnician, who helped the young searcher not only during normal business hours but also during long night sessions, necessary for the long-lasting surgeries at the beginning.

Performing the experimental studies besides the duties for the patients was only possible with the help of my teacher and mentor in plastic surgery, Prof. Heinz Bohmert. He also was interested in lymphedema after breast surgery and axillary dissection. He taught me the "Thompson procedure" for arm lymphedema.

The introduction of reconstructive lymph vascular surgery in the clinical field was supported by the head of the Department of Surgery, Prof. Georg Heberer. The first lymphatic vessel transplantation was performed on June 23, 1980, at the Department of Surgery of the Ludwig Maximilian University of Munich, Campus Grosshadern.

A series of candidates for the doctor's degree worked on this project: Ch. Gabka, U. Goldmann, D. Saumweber, M. Kressel, and Stefanie Springer, to mention only some of them.

Also, foreign guest researchers contributed to experimental studies, like M. Kudla from Czech Republic, M. El-Shazly from Egypt, and S. Sepulveda from Chile.

I'd like to thank especially Prof. Andreas Frick, who supported the clinical work through all these years. He also worked experimentally together with Prof. Johannes Hoffmann on the implication of liposuction and lymphatic structures.

PD. Dr. J. Wallmichrath contributed thereafter valuably to the scientific establishing of the lymphatic to lymph node approach.

Colleagues at the Department of Nuclear Medicine like E. Kleinhans, D.Hahn, and M. Weiss contributed to the search for objectifying the results by nuclear medical methods.

At the Institute for Clinical Radiology, M. Notohamiprodjo was supporting MRI lymphography studies.

The contribution by Mrs. E. Hanesch for the drawings and by Mr. A. Steeger for the photographic work is highly appreciated.

I thank Springer Nature Publishing for the help in editing this book.

Contents

Abbreviations

CDT	Complete decongestive therapy
CT	Compression therapy
DB-9	Druckrey-Berlin-9
e-PTFE	Expanded polytetrafluoroethylene
HE	Haematoxylin eosin
LE	Long-Evans
LL	Lymphatic load
LMU	Ludwig Maximilian University
LTC	Lymphatic transport capacity
Ltx	Lymphatic vessel transplantation
MLD	Manual lymph drainage
MRI	Magnetic resonance imaging
SEM	Standard error of the mean
SLS	Secondary liposuction
TI	Transport index
Tx	Transplantation
QOL	Quality of life

1 Pathophysiology of Lymphedemas with Respect to Surgery

1.1 Pathophysiology of Fluid Content

One essential element with respect to pathophysiology of lymphedema respects the fluid transport mechanisms within the lymphatic system. Lymphedemas are caused by an imbalance between the lymphatic fluid, which has to be cleared within a tissue area, e.g., an extremity, and the possibilities to transport this amount fluid out of the same area. Foeldi introduced the terms of the lymphatic load (LL) and the lymphatic transport capacity (LTC) (Földi 1971, 1985, Földi and Földi 2006).

Under normal circumstances, the lymphatic transport capacity surmounts the lymphatic load by far (Fig. 1.1). Therefore, damages to the lymphatic vessels are often without clinical consequences. There exist however regions, like narrowings or bottlenecks of the lymphatic system, where minor damages may result in a relatively large restriction on the lymphatic transport capacity (LTC). These are, for example, the axilla, the inguinal region, and the inner aspect of the knee. Furthermore danger for development of lymphedema occurs in cases of a diminished number of lymph nodes and lymphatic vessels like aplasias and atresias which may be the case in some primary lymphedemas (Kubik 1975, 1989; Brunner 1969). The ability to transport lymph is furthermore diminished by aging processes, perivascular fibrosis caused by radiation (Rubin and Casarett 1968), and by infectious alteration of lymphatic vessels. The other variable, the lymphatic load (LL), will be increased by infections, increased influx after venous compression, or an enforced working load. A sudden onset of lymphedema may be seen therefore years after the original trauma.

The pathophysiologic concept of the diminished transport (LTC) as origin for lymphedema leads to the surgical concept to overcome the diminished transport due to a localized lymphatic narrowing using a bypass procedure, an established method within vascular surgery (Fig. 1.2).

1.2 Pathophysiology of Non-soluble Contents

Imbalance between input and output of fluid is the primary origin of lymphedema. The disturbed function thereafter causes an alteration of the tissue composition within the affected area. Long time, mainly fibrotic tissue changes were mentioned as result of lymph stasis (Földi 1985; Földi and Földi 2006). However, the growth of fat tissue too was recognized as consequence of the lymph stasis. It is thought that lymphedema encourages lipid uptake (Ryan 1995).

The importance of fat was underlined by the clinical findings in long-standing lymphedema after decongestive treatment which showed almost only adipose tissue when collecting the suctioned material during treatment in lymphedema (Brorson and Svensson 1997).

Open surgical resection treatment procedures focus on the surplus of tissue and improve the shape of the edematous part by wide resections, including the skin, subcutaneous tissue, and optionally the fascia.

Modern strategies remove the surplus of adipose tissue by less-invasive methods like liposuction. The underlying disturbance of the fluid management of the lymphatic system is not corrected. Therefore recurrence has to be prevented by wearing elastic stockings continuously (Brorson and Svensson 1998).

Taking into account the vascular surgical option, it is possible to respecting the different aspects of lymphatic pathophysiology. This means first to restore the diminished lymphatic transport capacity, using the patient's own lymphatic vessels as graft, and second to resect the accumulated adipose tissue with the help of lymphatic vessel-sparing liposuction, if necessary and wished by the patient. This specific type of liposuction means that suctioning is only performed in longitudinal direction within an extremity, parallel to the direction of the main lym-

R.G.H. Baumeister, *Reconstructive Lymph Vascular Surgery*, DOI 10.1007/978-3-319-31647-5_1

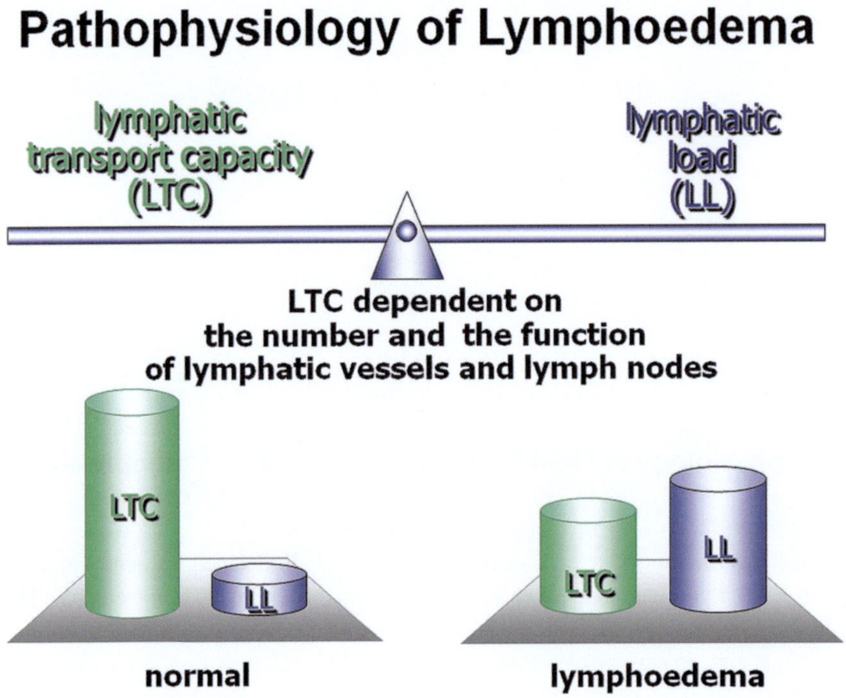

Fig. 1.1 Balance and imbalance of lymphatic fluid

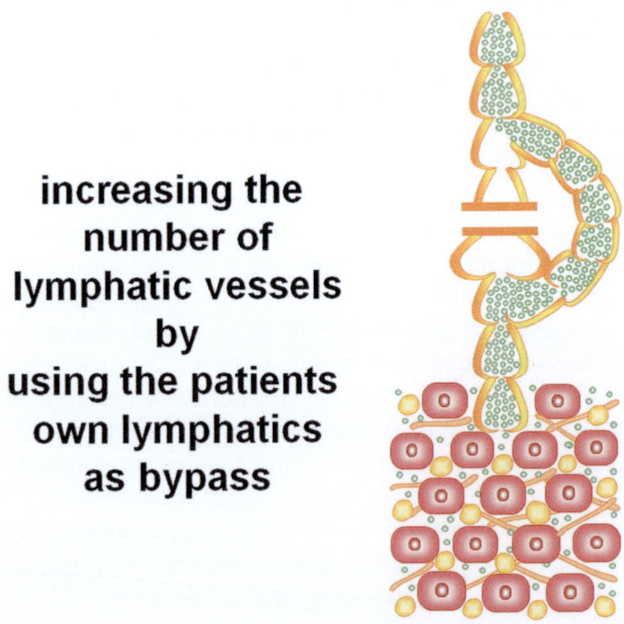

Fig. 1.2 Correcting the diminished lymphatic flow by a lymphatic bypass

phatic collectors. Extensive experimental studies have shown only minimal risk for the lymph vessels using the lymphatic vessel-sparing technique, especially in combination with a wet technique (Frick et al. 1999, 2006; Hoffmann et al. 2004).

References

Brorson H, Svensson H (1997) Complete reduction of lymphoedema of the arm by liposuction after breast cancer. Scan J Plast Reconstr Hand Surg 31:137

Brorson H, Svensson H (1998) Liposuction combined with controlled compression therapy reduces arm lymphedema more effectively than controlled compression therapy alone. Plast Reconstr Surg 102:1058

Brunner U (1969) Das Lymphödem der unteren Extremitäten. Hans Huber, Bern

Földi M (1971) Physiologie des Lymphgefäßsystems. Angiologica 8:212–235

Földi M (1985) The pathophysiology of lymphedema-insufficiency of the lymphvascular system. In: Bollinger A, Partsc H, Wolfe JHN (eds) The initial lymphatics. Thieme, Stuttgart, pp 2–6

Földi M, Földi E (2006) Physiology and pathophysiology of the lymphatic system. In: Földi M, Földi E (eds) Földi's textbook of lymphology, 2nd edn. Elsevier, Munich, pp 179–222

Frick A, Hoffmann JN, Baumeister RGH, Putz R (1999) Liposuction technique and lymphatic lesions in lower legs – an anatomical study to reduce its risks. Plast Reconstr Surg 103:1868–1873

Frick A, Baumeister RGH, Hoffmann JN (2006) Liposuction technique and lymphatics. In: Shiffmann MA, Di Guiseppe A (eds) Liposuction principles and practice. Springer, Heidelberg, pp 26–29

Hoffmann JN, Baumeister RGH, Fertmann J, Putz R, Frick A (2004) Tumescent an dry liposuction of lower extremities: differences in lymph vessel injury. Plast Reconstr Surg 113:718–724

Kubik S (1975) Zur klinischen Anatomie des Lymphsystems. Verh Anat Ges 69:109–116

Kubik S (1989) Anatomie des Lymphgefäßsystems. In: Földi M, Kubik S (eds) Lehrbuch der Lymphologie. Gustav Fischer, Stuttgart, pp 1–184

Rubin PH, Casarett GW (1968) Clinical radiation pathology. Saunders, Philadelphia

Ryan TJ (1995) Lymphatics and adipose tissue. Clin Dermatol 13:493–498

Experimental Basis of Reconstructive Lymph Vascular Surgery

2

2.1 Experiments and Training in Rats

Also experienced microsurgeons need additional training to work with lymphatic vessels.

The rat model, which is commonly used for microsurgical training, is also useful to become familiar with lymphatic vessels.

Furthermore, for starting an individual experience in dealing with lymphatic collectors, this experimental model is easily accessible and can give answer to the level of the personal success rate for anastomosing lymphatic vessels.

Also for establishing the technique, the rat model was used to evaluate basic strategies in lymphatic vessel microsurgery.

2.1.1 Training to Suture Lymphatic Vessels on the Abdominal Thoracic Duct

For the first attempts of training, the abdominal thoracic duct may be appropriate.

Under general anesthesia, the rat, with an optimal weight of about 250 g, is fixed lying on the back. The abdomen is opened via an incision beneath the left costal margin or a midline incision. The intestine together with the spleen is rotated to the right side and fixed with broad hooks (Fig. 2.1). With the help of two Q-tips, which are rotated in contrary direction, the aorta is exposed.

Just next to the aorta, the lymphatic abdominal thoracic duct is found on the left side. After a meal, the duct is seen as a milky structure filled with chyle. Otherwise it is recognized more difficulty just as a translucent structure.

The abdominal thoracic duct commences with the confluence of the lumbar and intestinal lymphatic ducts. On the way toward the diaphragm, it crosses the lumbar branches of the aorta. These should not get damaged because of possible bleeding. In between two branches, however, the abdominal thoracic duct is easily accessible (Fig. 2.2).

In direction to the diaphragm, care has to be taken not to open it accidentally since a pneumothorax will result.

The thoracic duct is separated from the aortic wall in a blunt technique with gentle movements by closed forceps. The border toward the abdominal aorta becomes obvious, and a similar procedure can be performed from the opposite side of the vessel.

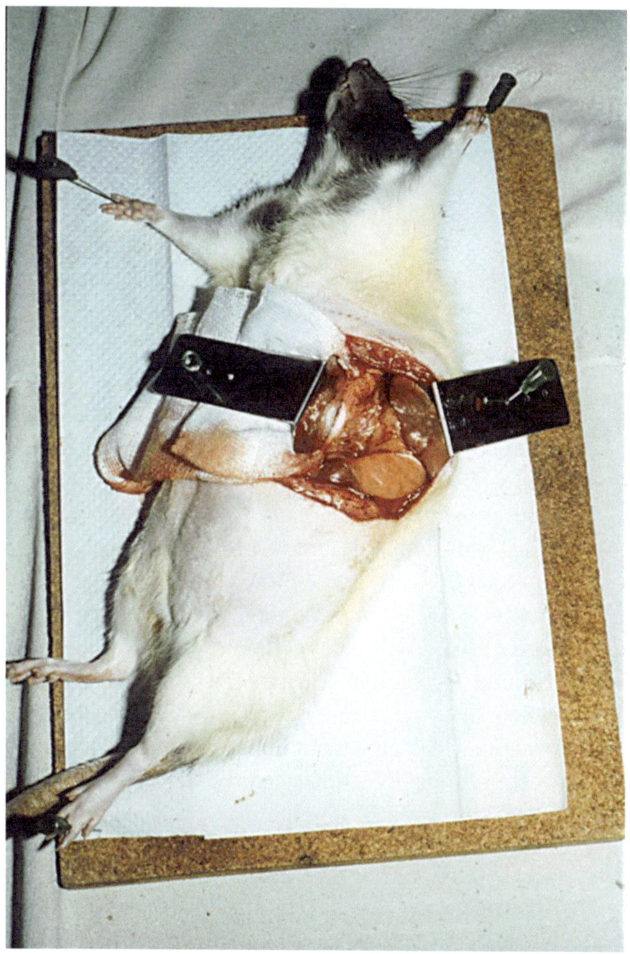

Fig. 2.1 Rat weighting around 250 g, the intestine together with the spleen is rotated to the right side and fixed with broad hooks; the left side of aorta is exposed

R.G.H. Baumeister, *Reconstructive Lymph Vascular Surgery*, DOI 10.1007/978-3-319-31647-5_2

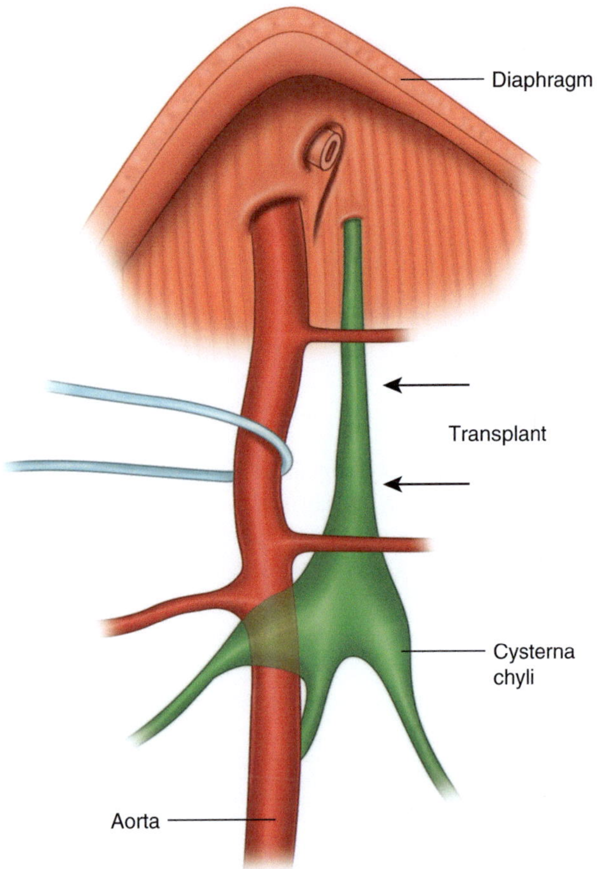

Fig 2.2 Access to the abdominal thoracic duct between the cisterna chyli and diaphragm between two lumbar branches for suturing and harvesting lymphatic segments for transplanting

The longtime experience with lymphatic vessels showed that, despite the thin wall, the vessels are relative resistant against longitudinal tension forces. They can be pulled and transferred with gentle stress.

If however the vessels are opened and tension is applied to the vessel wall in oblique direction, the fragile wall is ruptured very easily.

Small vessels are often anastomosed using the technique of Cobbett (1967). With this technique, the vessel wall is turned around to facilitate the suturing of the back wall with the help of corner sutures which are put under tension during rotation. This turned out not useful in suturing lymphatic vessels, since the corner sutures, set under tension, ruptured the tiny wall. In longitudinal direction, however, the vessels as a whole are remarkable resistant against tension.

The so-called tension-free anastomosing technique minimizes the forces applied to the vessel wall in oblique direction. It starts with a corner suture opposite to the surgeon. The back wall then is just lifted as far as the needle needs space to fix the back wall on both sides with single stitches leaving the knot on the outer surface. By that way the vessel remains in place without being turned around. Suturing of the back wall is completed with the second corner stitch in front of the surgeon. The front wall is thereafter easily completed by single stitches (Figs. 2.3, 2.4, 2.5, and 2.6) (Baumeister et al. 1981a, b, c).

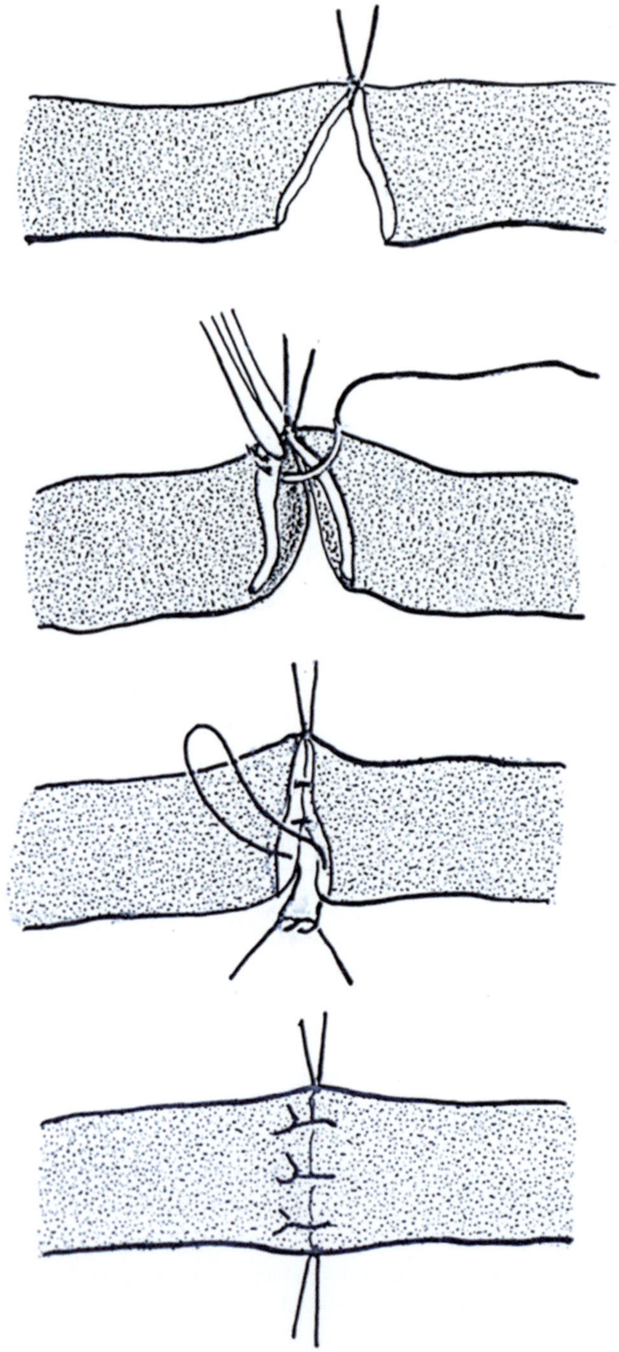

Fig. 2.3 Scheme of the "tension-free anastomosing technique," avoiding tension also in oblique direction starting with the first corner suture opposite to the surgeon, back wall gently lifted for single sutures, second corner suture and completing the front wall, no turning the vessel (With permission Baumeister et al. 1981 b from Wiley global permission)

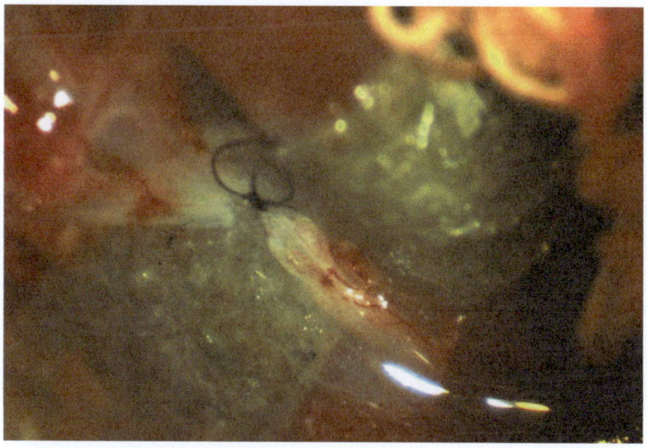

Fig. 2.4 First corner suture

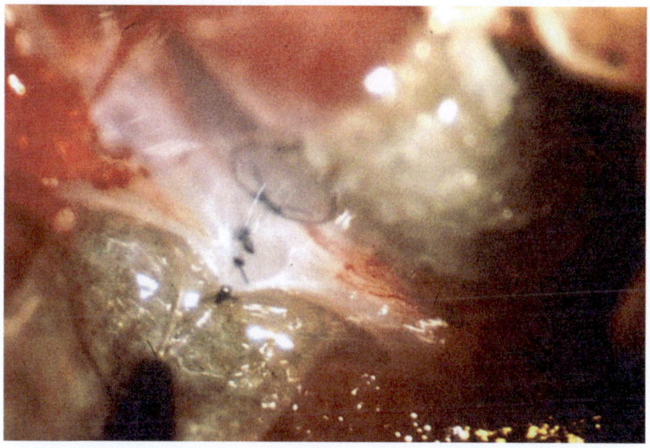

Fig. 2.5 Back wall completed as well as the second corner suture

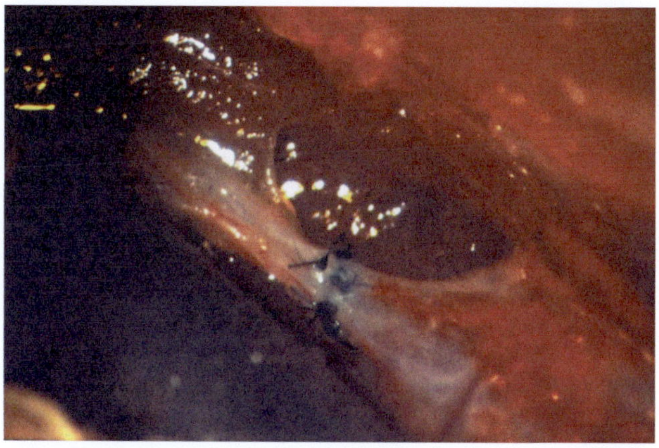

Fig. 2.6 Lymphatic vessel suture completed

For training, the vessel should not be transected completely at first since this would result in retraction of the two endings. The single stitches would have to be performed under tension. If however at least a small part of the wall remains, the suturing is possible without tension.

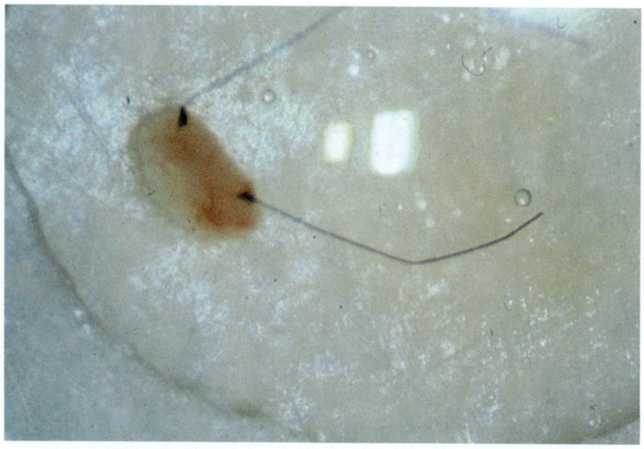

Fig. 2.7 Segment of the abdominal thoracic duct ready for grafting

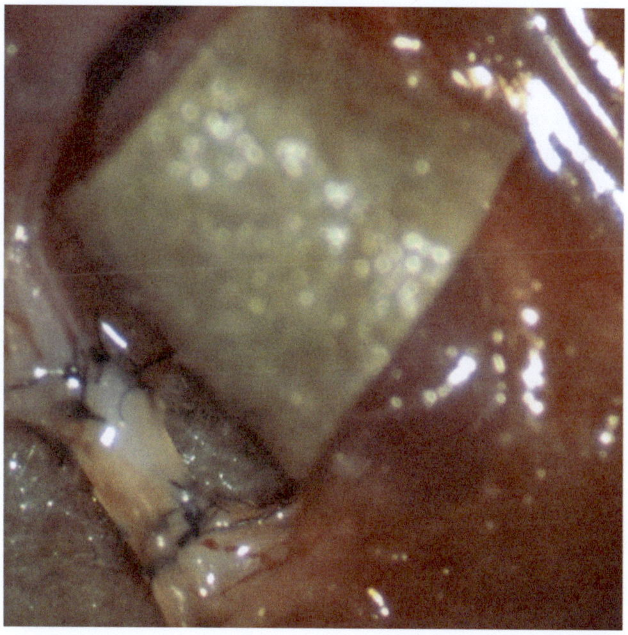

Fig. 2.8 Interposed lymphatic segment at the abdominal thoracic duct next to the rat aorta (With permission Baumeister et al. 1981b, from Wiley global permission)

In the case of a complete transection, it is recommended to interpose a lymphatic segment, harvested from a second animal. The interposed segment has to be inserted in the right direction of the lymphatic flow (Figs. 2.7 and 2.8).

It also gives the possibility to check the behavior of grafting in principle together with checking two anastomoses in a row.

For exercising, it might be useful to perform as many stitches as it might be applicable. However in man the number of sutures should be limited because the lymphatic vessels in patients are often much smaller than the abdominal thoracic duct in rats weighting 200–300 g.

With more experience, also the lumbar lymphatic vessels may be used for training to suture smaller lymphatic vessels.

2.1.2 Experiments on the Abdominal Thoracic Duct

2.1.2.1 Patency and Suture Material

At the abdominal thoracic duct, the patency of the anastomoses (Baumeister et al. 1980; 1981b), the patency rate of grafts (Baumeister et al. 1980; 1981b), and the reaction on the suture material (Baumeister et al. 1982a) were studied.

The patency was examined by visual examination after injection of dye (Patent Blue V®) and by histological examination. Patent Blue V® has a high molecular weight and is specifically taken in by the lymphatic capillaries.

Additionally, patency and function were studied using isotopes.

As atraumatic and monofilament suture material, absorbable polyglactin 910 (Vicryl®, Ethicon) and nonabsorbable Polyamide 6.6 ®, (Ethicon) size 10-0 to 12-0 were used.

After a mean observation period of 65 days, all ten grafts were judged as patent by inspection during the reoperation.

In 9 out of 10 grafts, the dye appeared cranial to the transplants after injection in the cisterna chyli.

Also 9 out of 10 grafts were proved patent by histological examination. In the occluded graft, nonabsorbable sutures have been used.

Out of the ten transplants, five were sutured with nonabsorbable Polyamide 6.6 and 5 with absorbable polyglactin 910 (Table 2.1).

During the whole investigation period, a marked foreign body reaction was seen around the nonabsorbable sutures (Fig. 2.9).

Table 2.1 Patency of autogenous lymphatic grafts in the rat abdominal duct

N=10	
Evaluation method	Patency
Inspection	10/10
Dye injection	09/10
Histology	09/10

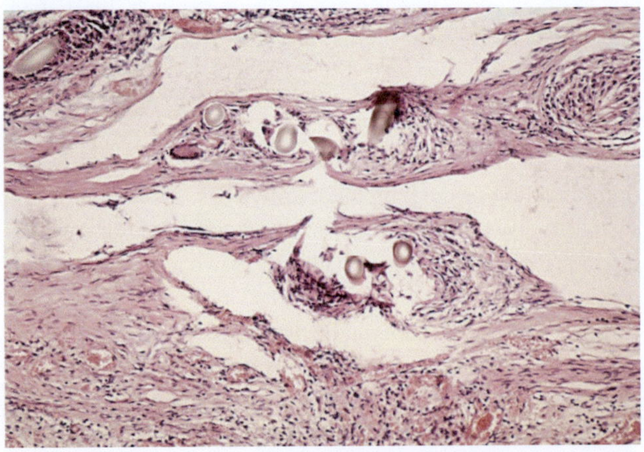

Fig. 2.9 Patent anastomosis of the abdominal thoracic duct, nonabsorbable suture material (Polyamide 6.6.), 8 weeks after surgery, marked foreign body reaction close to the vessel (H-E, tenfold magnification of objective)

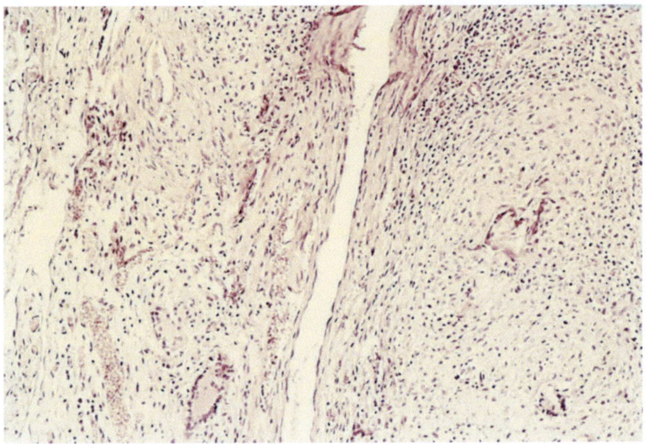

Fig. 2.10 Patent anastomosis of the abdominal thoracic duct, absorbable suture material polyglactin 910, 6 weeks after surgery, minor foreign body reaction (H-E, tenfold magnification of objective)

On the contrary, the reaction around the absorbable sutures diminished with time after the operation. Just remnants of the material were seen as contents of foreign body giant cells (Fig. 2.10).

In summary, the diameter of the foreign body reaction of the nonabsorbable material was bigger than the lymphatic vessel diameter itself. Therefore we used absorbable material further on. Polyglactin 910 was available with a size of 11-0 until the process of production was altered. Nowadays only the size 10-0 is available.

Lympho-lymphatic anastomoses have been investigated also by electron microscopy. Electron microscopy investigations revealed a smooth inner surface at the site of the anastomosis. In Fig. 2.11, the area of a lympho-lymphatic anastomosis is opened by an oblique cut of the vessel. The nonabsorbable suture material marks the site of the anastomosis. The vessel is stabilized by a small round insert for the electron microscopy preparation. The anastomosis is patent, the inner surface is smooth, and the endothelial layer is continued from one vessel to the other (Fig. 2.11).

2.1.2.2 Function of Grafts

Homologous transplantations of segments of the abdominal thoracic duct were performed on inbreeding Long-Evans and Lewis rats with an average weight of 250 g. The anastomoses were performed with the tension-free anastomosing technique.

The patency of the lymphatic grafts and the function as well were examined by injection of 131 I gamma globulin. The injection was performed within the cisterna chyli using an infusion pump. The activity was measured in the area above the thoracic duct in the chest (Fig. 2.12).

In untreated animals, a quick rise of activity could be observed after the injection. After ligation of the thoracic duct beneath the diaphragm, no elevated activity was detected at the chest. After interposition of the transplants, a quick rise in activity was seen like in normal animals (Fig. 2.13).

2.1.2.3 Immunologic Behavior of Transplanted Grafts

Grafts of the abdominal thoracic duct in a length of about 3 mm were harvested in Druckrey-Berlin 9 (DB9) rats, and they were interposed in the corresponding area in an orthodromic direction in Long-Evans (LE) rats.

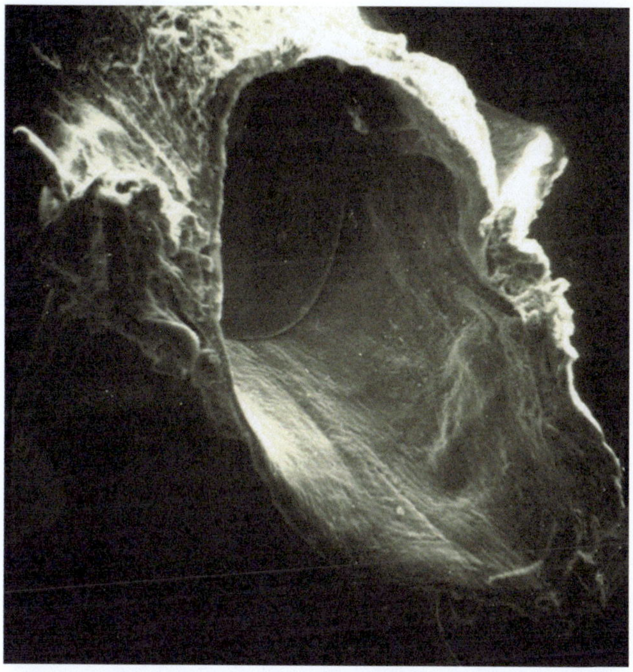

Fig 2.11 Scanning electron microscopy (oblique cut of the anastomosing site) 11 weeks after lympho-lymphatic anastomoses (nonabsorbable suture material), patent anastomosis, smooth inner surface continuous endothelial layer

In order to prove the genetic difference, in 10 DB9 animals, full-thickness skin grafts were transplanted with a diameter of 16 mm to Long-Evans rats. The grafted skin was rejected in 9 out of 10 animals at day 14, in one animal at day 16.

The results of the allogeneic transplantation were compared to the isogeneic transplantation in Long-Evans rats (Baumeister et al. 1982a, b; Gabka 1983).

The groups consisted of 15 animals.

The patency of the grafts was examined by inspection and by dye injections.

Random samples of the transplants were investigated also by electron microscopy.

After a mean observation period of 67 days, 14 out of 15 grafts were rated as patent by inspection and by dye injection in isogeneic transplantation.

In homologous transplantation, 13 out of 15 grafts were proved as patent after a mean follow-up period of 60 days (Table 2.2).

Between day 14 and 60 random investigations by electron microscopy were performed.

In normal abdominal thoracic ducts, the endothelium was smooth. The endothelial cells were closely connected, sometimes showing microvilli. Collagen fibers type I showed an exact arrangement in alternate directions. In between collagen fibers of type III were seen. Within the deeper layers of the lymphatic wall, fibrocytes, some capillaries, and single fat cells were seen.

In contrast, 14 days after allogeneic transplantation, no continuous endothelial covering could be detected. Instead, the inner surface was covered by a fibrous network. The formerly structured arrangement of collagen fibers was destructed. Collagen fibers type I and II were thus present on the inner surface.

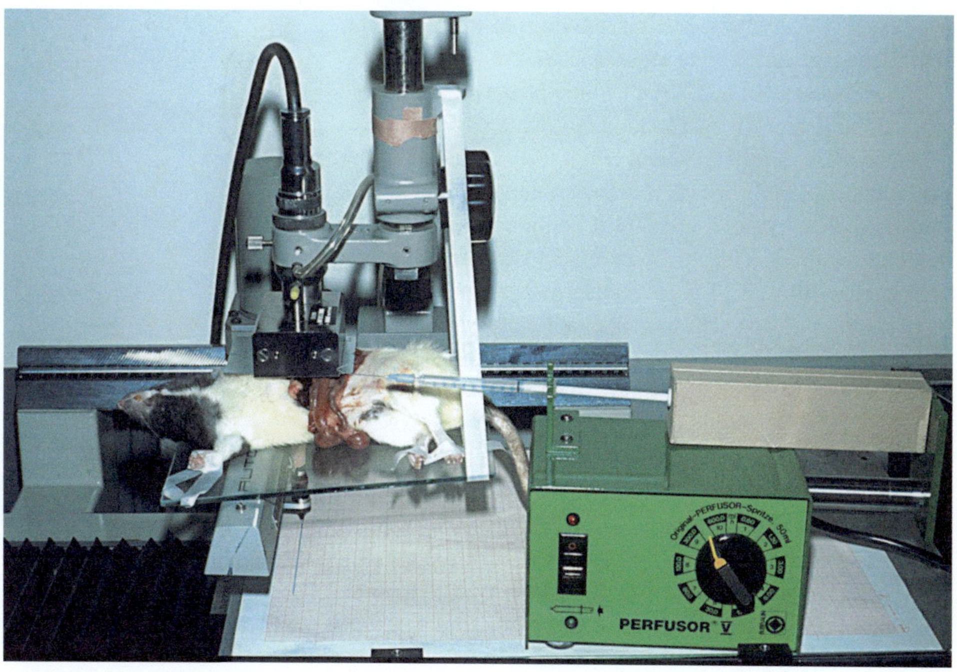

Fig. 2.12 Assessment of function after reconstruction of the abdominal thoracic duct by lymphatic grafts, injection of 131 I gamma globulin in the cisterna chyli, measurement above the thorax

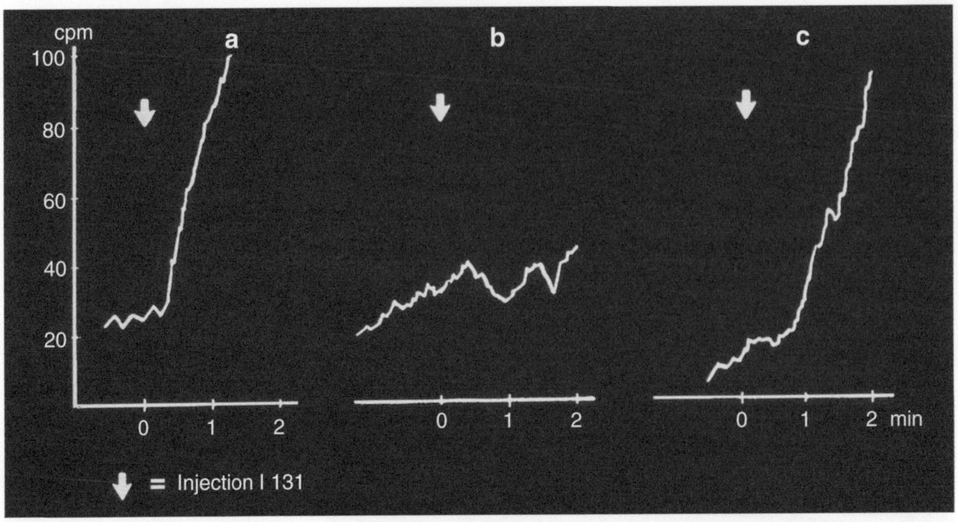

Fig. 2.13 Measuring the activity of marked albumin at the chest after injection into the cisterna chyli (*arrow*, start of the injection). (**a**) Untreated animal. (**b**) After ligation of the abdominal thoracic duct beneath the diaphragm. (**c**) 8 weeks after transection of the abdominal thoracic duct and interposing a lymphatic graft (*arrow*, Injektionsbeginn: starting the injection) (With permission Baumeister et al. 1981b, from Wiley global permission)

Table 2.2 Patency of isogeneic and allogeneic transplanted segments of the abdominal thoracic duct in rats

	Isogeneic transplantation	Allogeneic transplantation
Evaluation method	Mean observation period 67 days	Mean observation period 60 days
Inspection	14/15	13/15
Dye injection	14/15	13/15

Within blood-containing vessels, the collagen fibers type III would increase the risk of thrombosis. In lymphatic vessels, however, no significant thrombosis was seen. The reason for this might be that the potential of coagulation is reduced in lymphatic fluid to about one-third, and therefore no thrombosis was detected (Yoffey and Courtice 1970).

During weeks 3 and 4, a neointima started from the adjoining intact duct to cover the whole inner surface of the transplants. Blood capillaries grow in the vessel wall toward the neointima.

Between days 40 and 60, within the wall caverns appeared, together with a massive infiltration of activated lymphocytes, plasma cells, macrophages, and erythrocytes. The wall however remained stable because of the new endothelium and the subendothelial tissue containing a continuous basal membrane, structured collagen fibers type I, and differentiated muscle cells (Figs. 2.14, 2.15, and 2.16).

In summary, allogeneic transplantation of segments of the abdominal thoracic duct from DB9 rats to LE rats showed a high long-term patency rate similar to that seen in isogeneic transplantation. Investigation by electron microscopy showed an immunologic reaction, first at the endothelium and later in the deeper areas of the vessel wall. This did however not cause a destruction of the transplant and interfere with the function. The low pressure within the lymphatic transporting system and the low coagulability of lymphatic fluid might be the reasons for these surprising findings.

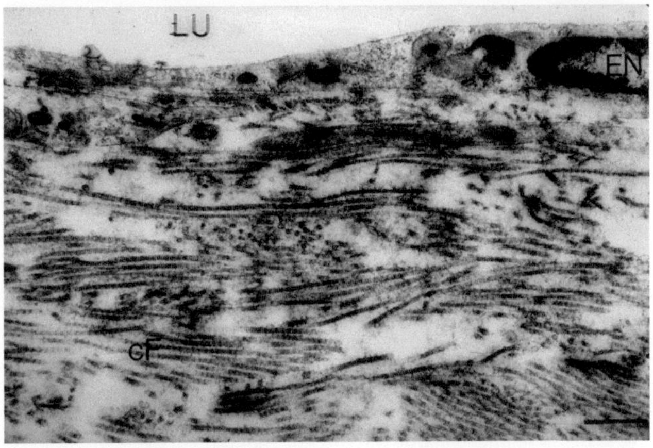

Fig. 2.14 Allogeneic abdominal thoracic duct graft of rat. 40 days after grafting (ultrathin section, 1000-fold magnification) (*E* endothelial cell, *LU* lumen, *cF* collagen fibers)

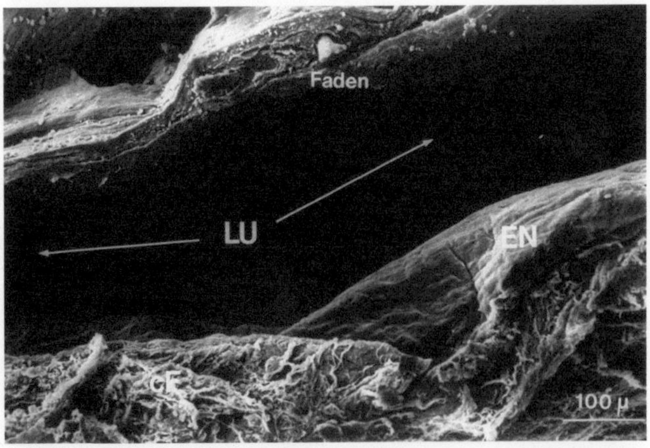

Fig. 2.15 Allogeneic abdominal thoracic duct graft of rat. 40 days after grafting (scanning electron microscopy, 440-fold magnification). *LU* lumen, *EN* endothelium, *cF* collagen fibers, *Faden* suture)

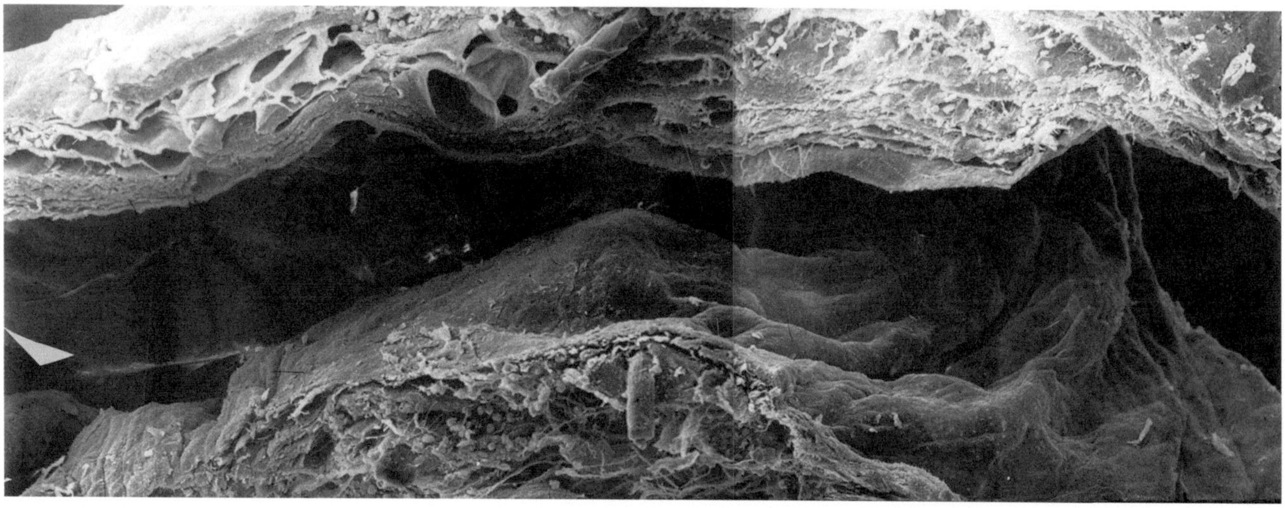

Fig. 2.16 Allogeneic abdominal thoracic duct graft of rat 60 days after grafting (scanning electron microscopy, composition 700-fold magnification), site of anastomosis, graft left, host-vessel right

2.1.2.4 Storage of Lymphatic Grafts

Since experiments with allogeneic transplantation of lymphatic grafts revealed stable and functioning lymphatic transplant, the consequences of storage of the grafts were studied (Baumeister et al. 1983; Goldmann 1987).

Segments of the abdominal thoracic duct in Long-Evans rats with a length of 3 mm were stored in different media and different time periods.

For studying the patency, the grafts were subsequently interposed at the corresponding area of the recipient in the so-called tension-free anastomosing technique using monofilament polyglactin 910 sutures size 10 to 11-0.

The patency was examined by inspection and dye injection.

Additionally, lymphatic segments were investigated by scanning and transmission electron microscopy.

The short-time storage between 30 min and 10 h in 0.9 % NaCl solution at 4° and 20 °C revealed no structural changes within the vessel wall. The endothelial layer however became destructed with increased duration of storage, whereas the deep structures of the vessel wall remained intact. Figure 2.17 shows the intact endothelial layer after 30 min of storage in 0.9 % NaCl solution at 4 °C.

After a medium storage period of 8 days at 4 °C in 0.9 % NaCl solution, the endothelial sheet was disconnected. Partly cell lysis occurred. Also the subendothelial tissue showed a disintegration of collagen elements and a lysis of fibrocytes.

The short-term stored and subsequently transplanted grafts showed a patency in all ten animals, 20 days after grafting. All grafts showed a nearly complete endothelial lining.

After storage of 8 days, 2–40 days after surgery all grafts in the ten investigated animals were patent. Figure 2.18 shows a patent anastomosis (located at the upper edge of the figure), 2 days after grafting after a storage of 8 days at 4 °C examined by scanning electron microscopy with 120-fold magnification.

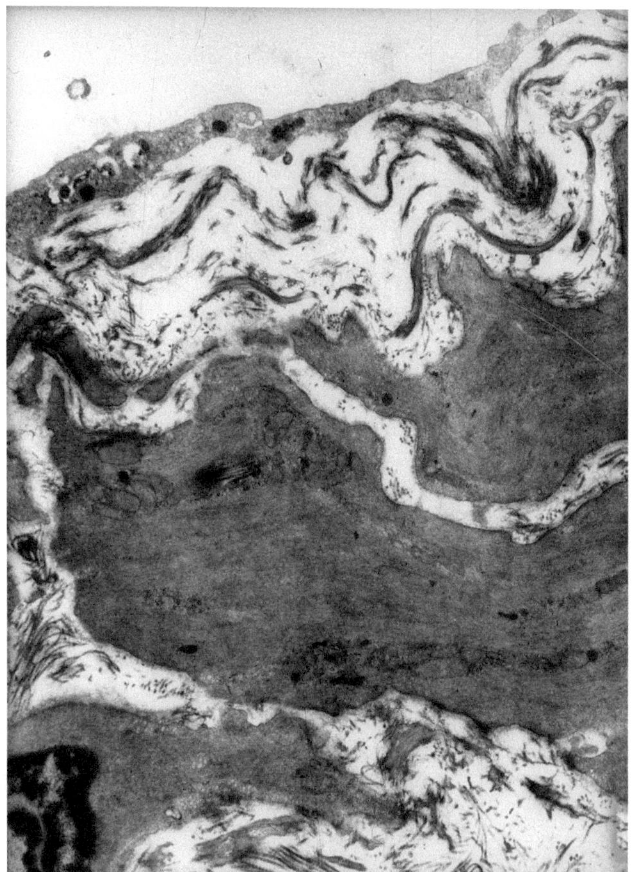

Fig 2.17 30 min storage in 0.9 % NaCl solution at 4 °C

The inner lining was built by fibrin at days 2 and 4. Between days 8 and 40, a complete endothelial layer again

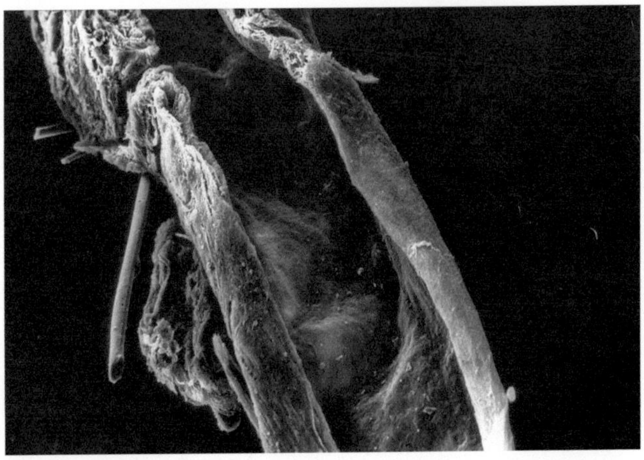

Fig. 2.18 Patent graft, 8 days of storage at 4 °C, 2 days after grafting

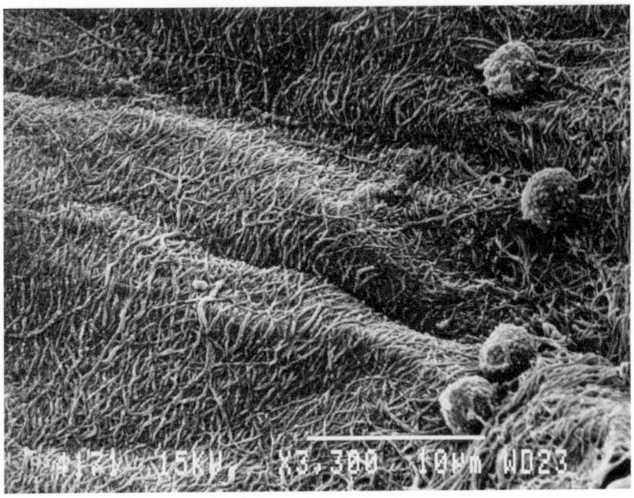

Fig 2.19 e-PTFE prosthesis 3 days after implantation, covered by a pseudointima built out of fibrin, with four lymphocytes (scanning electron microscopy, 3300-fold original magnification)

was seen. The subendothelial layer was restructured by collagen fibers. Between days 30 and 40, for the first time, muscle cells appeared.

After a storage period of 30 days, again all transplants in the three investigated animals were patent. There were no differences within the wall observed compared to the previous findings.

Using longer graft, however, like in the dog model, comparable results could not be achieved (see experiments in dogs)

In summary, as seen in allogeneic transplantation, the short lymphatic vessels remain open also after storage time at 4 °C up to 40 days. At least in short grafts, regeneration of the endothelium is possible, starting from adjacent normal vessels. Storage at 20 °C is less favorable, at least at longer storage times.

2.1.2.5 Replacement of Lymphatic Grafts by PTFE Segments

Since in some patients harvesting of lymphatic grafts may be a problem, artificial material might have a place in reconstructive lymph vascular surgery. Therefore also studies including artificial material were performed (Saumweber et al. 1987, 1988; Saumweber 1989).

In 19 rats the resected abdominal thoracic duct was replaced by short e-PTFE micro-prostheses with a length of 4–5 mm. The follow-up period ranged between 2 and 335 days. 17 prostheses out of 19 were rated as patent by inspection and dye injection. 18 prostheses were judged patent in the investigation by electron microscopy.

With the use of longer e-PTFE grafts with a length of 5–6 mm, however, only in 3 out of 10 were rated as patent by clinical and histological examination at a follow-up period of 2–35 days. At day 2 all grafts were patent. From day 14 on, none of the grafts remained patent.

The electron microscopy revealed in the patent grafts a pseudointima, made out of a thin fibrin layer.

Figure 2.19 shows an e-PTFE prosthesis 3 days after implantation, covered by a pseudointima built out of fibrin, with four lymphocytes.

From day 7 on, a mostly complete endothelial layer with superficial and deep fibrous strata was seen. Later on capillaries and muscle cells appeared.

In the occluded grafts, first, a fibrin thrombus occluded the lumen. Later on fibrin tissue invaded the thrombus at several parts, whereas in other parts a normal wall was seen.

In contrast, the experiments in dogs with longer grafts did not show patent grafts (see experiments in dogs).

In summary, as seen in former studies about immunologic behavior and the effect of storage in short lymphatic grafts, also short artificial implants with a length of 4–5 mm remained patent and showed a regeneration of the endothelial layer. Implants with a length of 5–6 mm remained open only during a period of less than 14 days.

2.1.2.6 The Use of Lymphatic Grafts in Organ Transplantation

In organ transplantation, routinely only arteries and veins are reconstructed. The lymphatic vascular system however is forced to regenerate spontaneously. Therefore, at least during the first days exists a lack of lymphatic communication between graft and host.

This might be of utmost importance in small bowel transplantation. There, the importance of lymphatic tissue is obvious, especially with respect to the resorption of fat and the possible graft versus host reaction.

We developed a method for a combined anastomosing procedure of the three vascular systems in small bowel transplantation. The grafts were harvested in Sprague-Dawley rats together with the lymphatic vessels including the cisterna

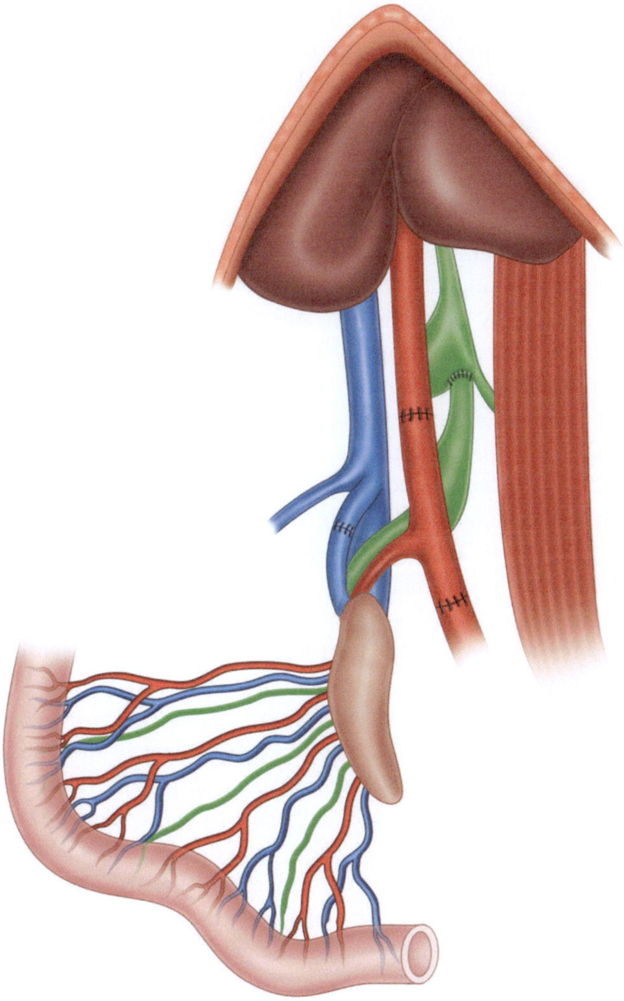

Fig. 2.20 Scheme of anastomoses of artery, vein, and lymphatic vessel in small bowel transplantation in rats

chyli and parts of the abdominal thoracic duct and the adjacent aorta together with the superior mesenteric artery and the portal vein (Kressel 1995).

In the host, anastomoses were performed with the aorta, the left renal vein, and the cisterna chyli (Figs. 2.20 and 2.21).

In a first study with 5 animals, patency was proved in 4 rats using a water-soluble contrast medium (Isovist®) and radiological controls.

Regarding survival rate and technical complication in a series of 17 rats, five animals were lost mostly due to technical reasons within the first 5 days. 12 animals were followed for 1–2 weeks, when a slow rejection did occur due to genetic differences in this brand of animals.

One effect of an additional primary repair of the lymphatic vessels should be an improvement in resorption of long-chained fatty acids especially in the first days.

Without primary repair, spontaneous regeneration at some extent takes at least 7–10 days, which affects absorption of

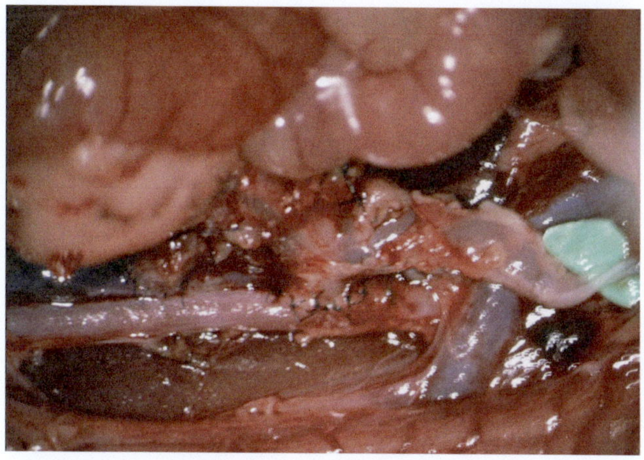

Fig. 2.21 Anastomoses of artery, vein, and lymphatic vessel in small bowel transplantation in rats

fat and fat-soluble molecules such as cyclosporine (Wood and Ingham Clark 1991).

We administered the long-chained fatty acid, 15(S)-hydroxy-5,8,11,13-eicosatetraenoic acid (15 HETE), at days 8, 21, and 50 via the transplanted small bowel.

Blood samples were taken before administering and after 30, 60, 90, and 120 min.

A higher level of the measured long-chained fatty acid at day 8 was seen in animals with primary lympho-lymphatic repair compared to animals in which only artery and vein have been anastomosed (Sepulveda et al. 1994).

Immediate contact between graft and host in small bowel transplantation under therapy using cyclosporine A treatment might therefore have also an influence in graft survival.

In allogeneic small bowel transplantation, primary reconstruction of the lymphatic vessels resulted, according to our preliminary results, in an avoidance of acute allograft rejection under a short-term cyclosporine A treatment (Szymula von Richter and Baumeister 1998).

2.1.2.7 Lymphatic to Lymph Node Anastomoses

Another way of direct reconstruction of an interrupted lymphatic transporting system is to connect the lymphatic grafts to lymph nodes.

In the clinical field, this is important for the cranial anastomoses in treatment of arm edema. Sometimes it is easier to connect the graft directly to the nodes, especially at a region where the lymphatic vessels themselves are thin and lymph nodes are present in a higher number.

In rats, at the lumbar area, there are lymphatic channels as well as lymph nodes present on each side of the big vessels. This gives the possibility to use one side for harvesting and the other side for anastomosing (Figs. 2.22 and 2.23).

The preparation is facilitated if dye (Patent Blue V®) is administered beforehand on the side of harvesting. The

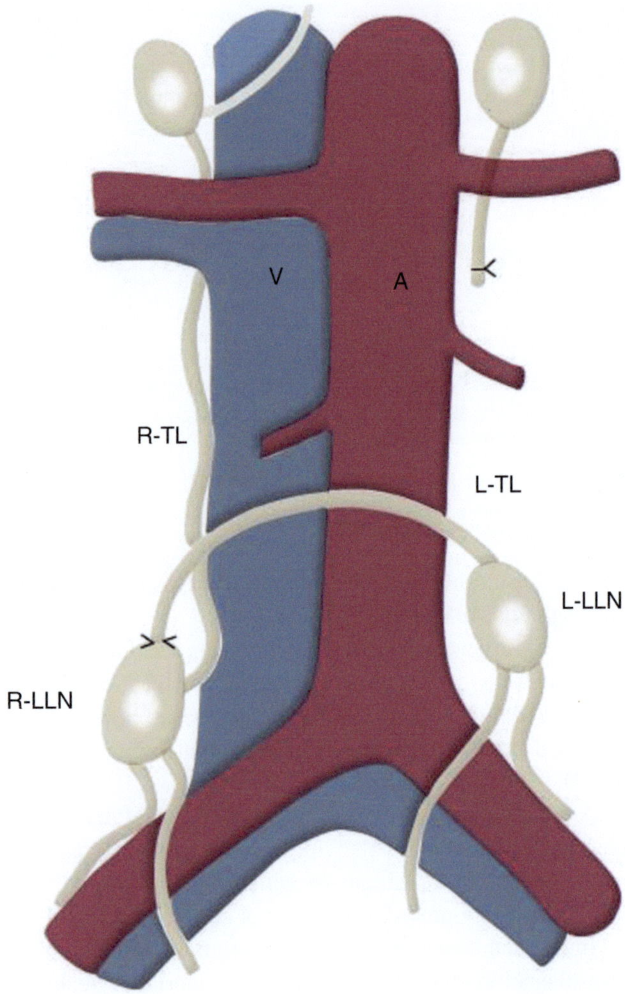

Fig. 2.22 Schematic drawing of the lympho-lymphonodular anastomoses: the left lumbar trunk above the lymph nodes of the left side is transposed to the opposite side and anastomosed to the lymph node at the right side

lumbar trunk then is better to distinguish. The lymph nodes on the opposite side are exposed without staining.

The lymphatic lumbar trunk is then divided far proximally to get enough length for transposing the vessels to the opposite side.

On the lymph nodes, next to the effluent vessel, the capsule is opened superficially not to damage the deeper structures and generate bleeding according to the diameter of the transposed lymphatic vessel. The outer sinuses should just be opened. A bleeding indicates that damages to deeper structures did occur (Fig. 2.23).

In order to establish the technique and prove the patency rate, experiments in rats have been performed (Wallmichrath et al. 2011) (Fig. 2.24).

The lymphatic structures at the pelvis with the right and left lumbar routes, containing lymphatic vessels and lymph nodes as well, allow using one side for harvesting and the other side for anastomosing.

16 Sprague-Dawley rats were investigated.

After staining with Patent Blue V, in eight animals, the left lumbar trunk was cut cranially. The distal part was turned over to the right side. There, at the lymph node, a small part of the capsule was excised distant to the hilus, corresponding to the diameter of the transposed lymphatic vessel. Care was taken not to damage the well-vascularized marrow of the lymph node. This procedure avoids bleeding and gives direct access to the superficial sinuses. The anastomosis was performed in a tension-free single-stitch technique using absorbable suture material (polyglactin 910). The posterior wall was sutured first. Each stitch started at the surface of the lymph node. Two to four stitches were used per anastomosis. In two animals, a doubled lymphatic trunk was found at the left side and two anastomoses were performed.

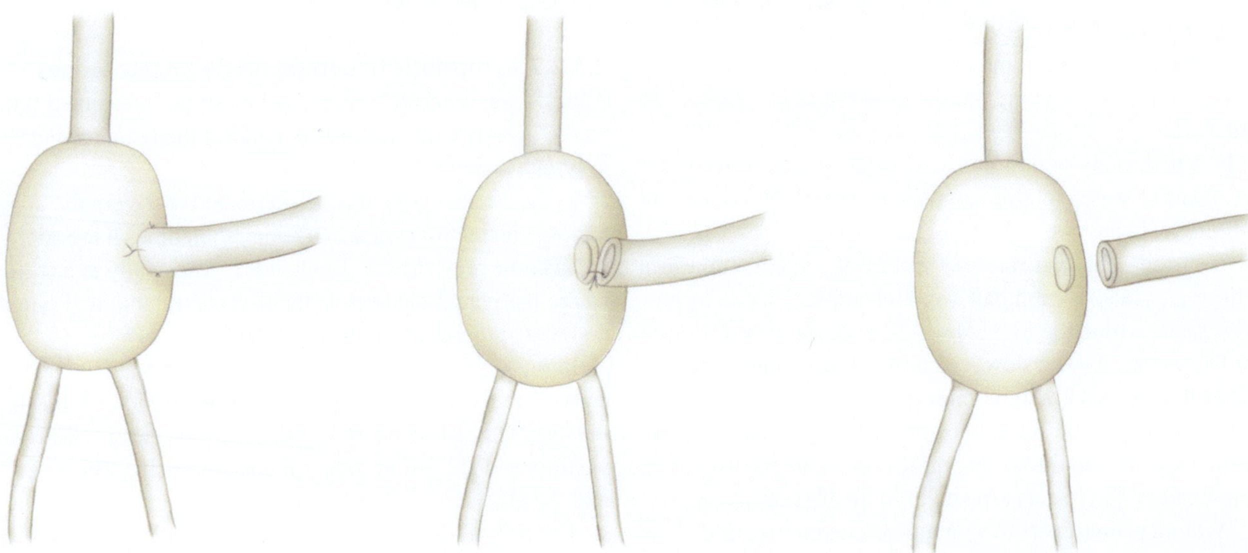

Fig. 2.23 Microsurgical procedure for a lympho-lymphonodular anastomoses. The graft is anastomosed to an appropriate excision of the capsule of the lymph node

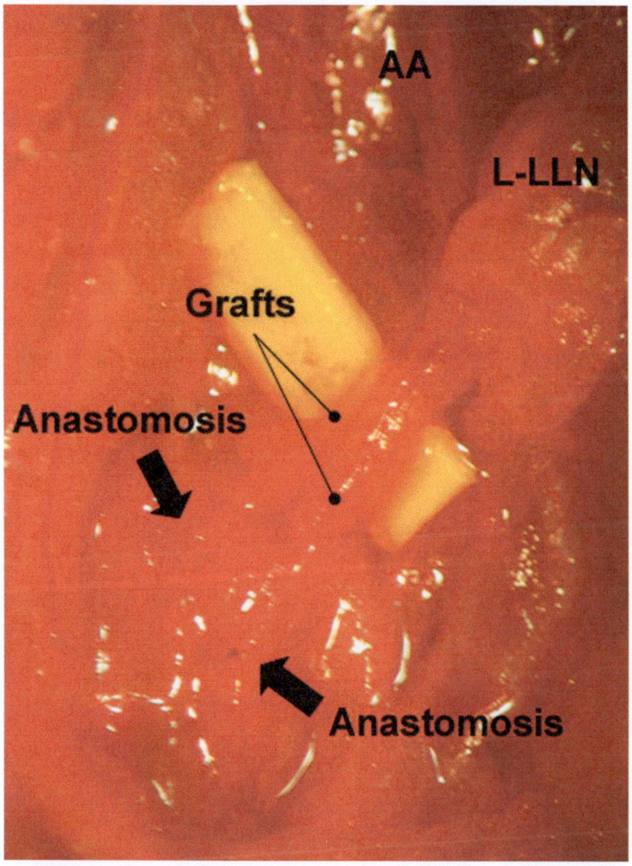

Fig. 2.24 Intraoperative picture of lympho-lymphonodular anastomosis between a lymphatic vessel departing from a left lumbar lymph node, transversing the aorta and anastomosed to the right lumbar lymph node (Courtesy PD Dr. Wallmichrath)

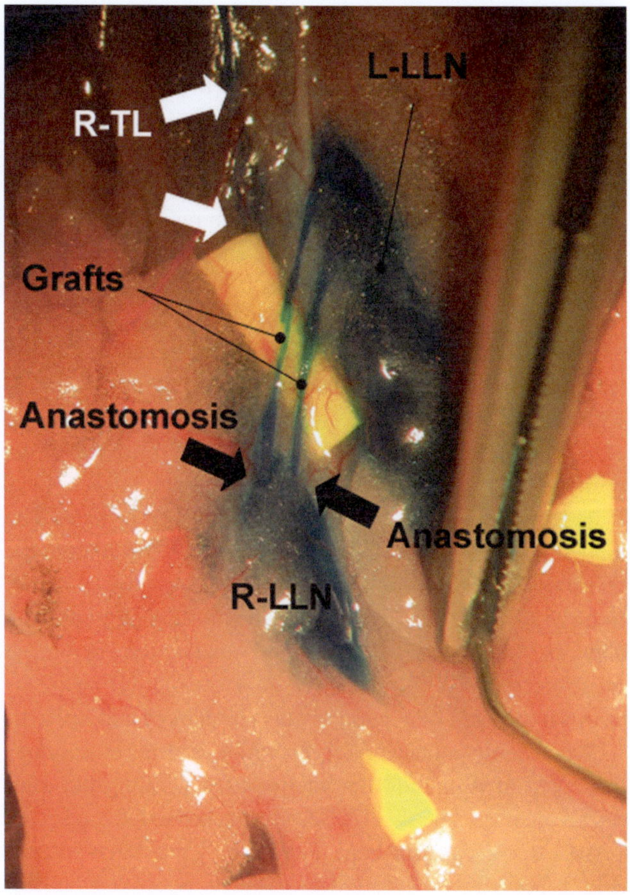

Fig. 2.25 Proved patency of lympho-lymphonodular anastomosis, stained grafts, and stained right lymph node after injection of Patent Blue V ® in the left lumbar lymph node (Courtesy PD Dr. Wallmichrath)

In eight controls the left lumbar lymphatic trunk was cut and ligated.

The patency was proved after a follow-up period of 8 weeks by observation of a free transit of the dye and indirectly by observation of a staining of the connected lymph nodes.

In the anastomosis group, 8 out of 8 animals showed patent anastomoses and regular outflow to the right lumbar system.

In the group without transposing lymphatic vessels in 6 out of 8 animals, no lymphatic connection to the right lumbar lymphatic system was seen.

The difference between the two groups was significant (Wallmichrath et al. 2009).

In a second study consisting of 36 Sprague-Dawley rats, the difference was examined between a direct lympho-lymphonodular anastomosis and a possible spontaneous lympho-lymphonodular anastomosis.

In 12 rats lymphatic vessels from the left lumbar trunk were transposed to the opposite side and microsurgical lympho-lymphonodular anastomoses were performed as described above.

In 12 rats the lymphatic vessels were transposed but no anastomoses were performed.

In a third group of 12 rats, the left lumbar trunk was transected; there was no transposing of the vessel. The capsule of the lymph node at the right side was only incised.

After 8, 12, and 16 weeks, the lumbar region were explored and the way of Patent Blue V followed after peripheral injection at the left paw.

In 12 out of 12 animals of the anastomosing group, patent transposed lymphatic vessels and anastomoses with blue staining of the right lymph node were seen (Fig. 2.25).

1 out of 12 animals with transposed lymphatic vessels, however without opening the lymph nodes capsule, showed a blue staining of the right lymph node. In the group without transposing lymphatic vessels to the opposite side, but an opening the lymph node capsule at the contralateral side, 2 out of 12 rats showed a stained lymph node at the right side (Wallmichrath et al. 2012).

The results showed that anastomosing between lymphatic vessels and lymph nodes is possible and reveals a high patency. This is in contrast to spontaneous lympho-lymphonodular anastomosing which does not occur.

2.2 Experiments in Dogs

2.2.1 The Experimental Canine Model

To prove the efficiency of lymphatic vessel grafting in treating lymphedemas, a bigger animal model was necessary. In the literature different models have been reported. The main problem consists of the spontaneous anastomosing ability of the lymphatic system which makes it difficult to establish a permanent edema.

We used the lymphedema model of the hind leg of the dog which was described by Clodius and Wirth (1974, 1977) with some modifications.

In general anesthesia, the dog is lying in a back-prone position.

In the middle of the thigh, a circular incision is made. The hind limb is then totally transected except the femur, the femoral artery, the vein, and the nerve and the ischial nerve. In order to clean the vessels from all surrounding lymphatic network, this part is performed under the operating microscope.

All transected lymphatic vessels are marked and ligated.

To prevent spontaneous regeneration, a sheet of polyurethane/Teflon (Epigard®) is interposed, separating the transected muscles. The sheet is closely attached to the transected vessels, nerves, and the bone. Finally, only the skin is sutured (Fig. 2.26).

This procedure leads to a total blockade of the deep and superficial lymphatic system. The weakest part is the skin since the suture line is not enforced by the underlying tissue.

The lymphedema is fully developed after about 1 week (Fig. 2.27).

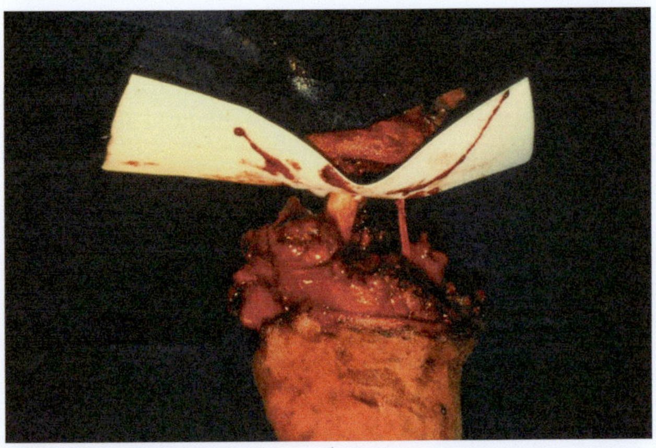

Fig. 2.26 Experimental lymphedema of the hind leg in dogs according to Clodius and Wirth, prevention of lymphatic regeneration by an interposed polyurethane/Teflon barrier (With permission Baumeister et al. 1981b, from Wiley global permission)

2.2.2 Treating Experimental Lymphedema by Lymphatic Grafts

The contralateral limb serves thereafter as harvesting area. Within the subcutaneous tissue, lymphatic collectors at the medial thigh are used as grafts. First, the dye (Patent Blue V®) is injected subcutaneously at the paw. Passive movements facilitate the transport in direction to the groin region. After some minutes the stained lymphatic collectors can be found easily. Two to three of them are dissected at the thigh and used thereafter as grafts at the edematous leg (Fig. 2.28).

At the edematous limb, the lymphatic vessels are dissected peripheral and central to the barrier in preparation of the reconstruction.

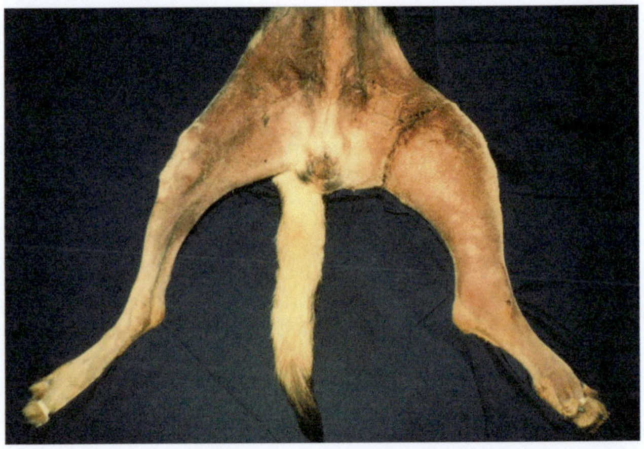

Fig. 2.27 Experimental lymphedema of hind leg in the dog due to local blockade at the thigh (With permission Baumeister et al. 1981c, from Springer)

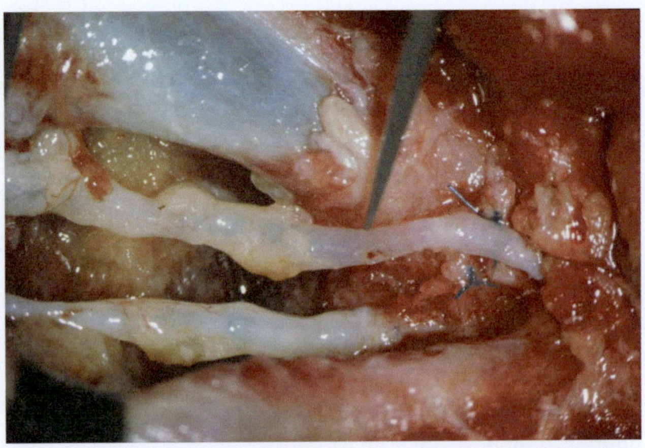

Fig. 2.28 Two lymphatic vessel grafts reconstructing the interrupted lymphatic vessels

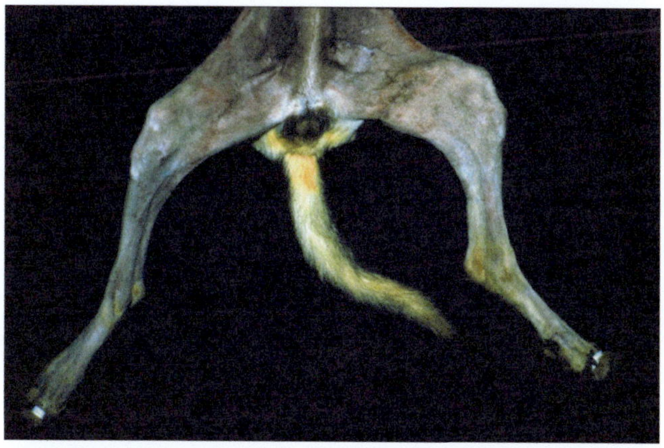

Fig. 2.29 Return to normal seize, 4 weeks after lymphatic transplantation (With permission Baumeister et al. 1981c, from Springer)

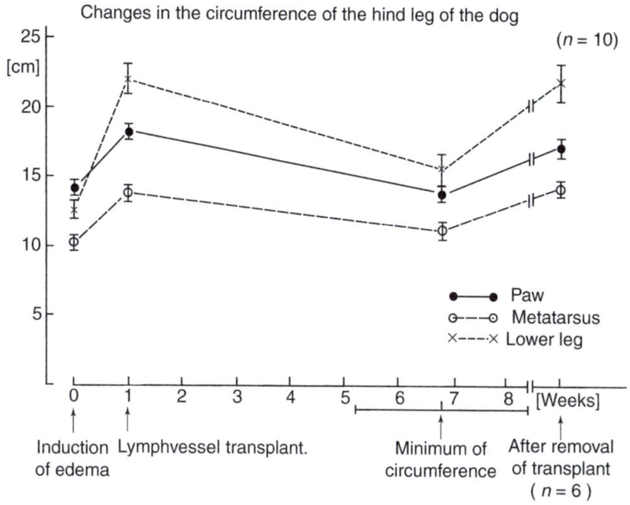

Fig. 2.30 Significant changes in the circumference at the hind leg after inducing a lymphedema, after reconstruction by lymphatic grafts, and after removal of the graft (measurements at the paw, metatarsus, and lower leg in ten dogs)

The grafts are anastomosed in the tension-free anastomosing technique. Under the operating microscope, the first stitch is performed opposite to the surgeon. The back wall is sewn with interrupted sutures thereby the wall being lifted only enough to allow the needle to pass. The anastomosis is finished with interrupted sutures at the front wall. Throughout the whole anastomosing procedure, no tension in oblique direction occurs. Polyglactin 910 size 10-0 to 11-0 was used in the original experiments. The size 11-0 was available at the time of the investigation, whereas at the present time, only 10-0 polyglactin 910 suture material is available.

After a follow-up period of about 7 weeks after lymphatic reconstruction, the circumferences diminished significantly and reached normal values (Fig. 2.29).

Circumferences were measured at the paw, the metatarsus, and the lower leg. After producing the edema, a significant increase was seen. When the grafts have been removed, the circumferences again raised significantly (Fig. 2.30).

2.2.3 Patency of Grafts

After a period of about 7 weeks, the edema had disappeared, and the operating field was opened in the search for the transplanted collectors and the anastomoses.

The patency was investigated in ten dogs with a mean follow-up period of 50 days.

First the patency was proved by visual inspection without and with peripheral dye (Patent Blue V ®) administering. The patency was stated if at least one graft in the animal was seen patent (Figs. 2.31 and 2.32).

Furthermore, the patency of the grafts was proved by direct lymphography using the oily contrast medium (Lipiodol Utrafluid®). The lymphatic graft had to be demon-

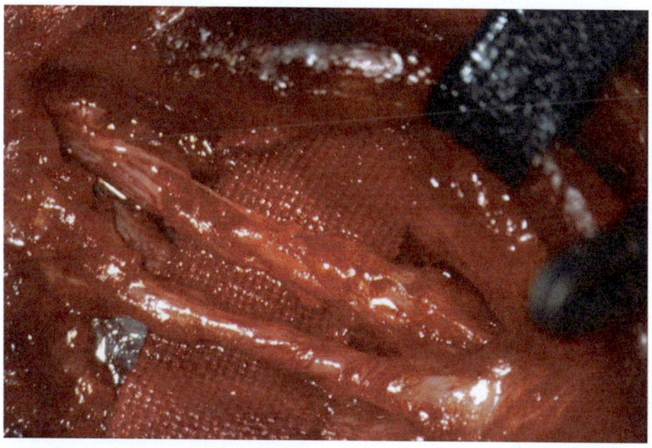

Fig. 2.31 Reexploration of transplanted lymphatic vessels, 4 weeks after grafting (With permission Baumeister et al. 1981c, from Springer)

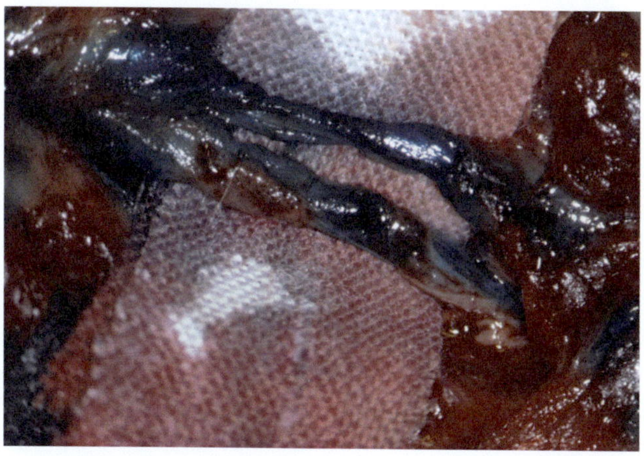

Fig. 2.32 Proof of patency of lymphatic grafts, stained grafts after peripheral injection of dye (Patent Blue V ®)

strated radiologically within two metallic markers which were located in front and behind areas of grafting (Fig. 2.33).

Administering isotopes (131 I gamma globulin) at the paw revealed patency and function as well when activity was detected at the groin.

Finally the specimens were examined histologically.

In 8 out of 10 dogs, the patency was demonstrated by inspection, lymphography, and isotopes.

In all ten animals proof of patency was possible with the help of histological examination (Table 2.3).

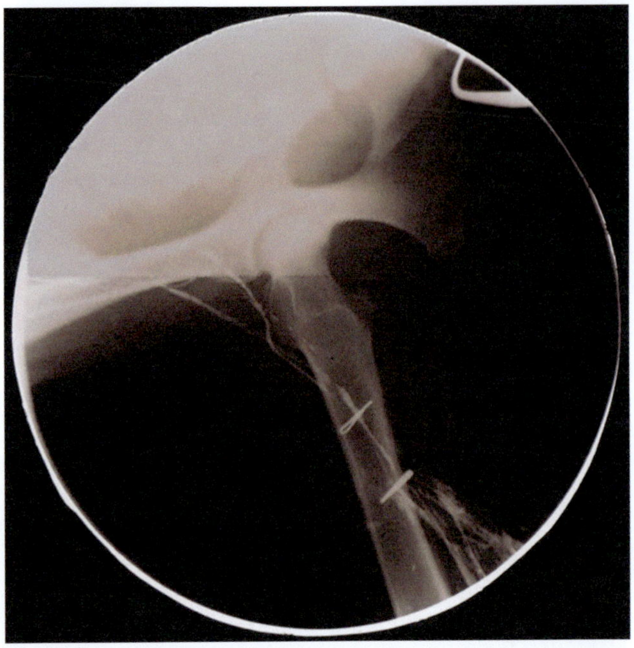

Fig. 2.33 Proof of patent lymphatic grafts by oily contrast medium (Lipiodol®), seen between the markers distal and proximal to the areas of grafting

Table 2.3 Patency of lymphatic grafts in the experimental lymphedema of dogs

Evaluation method	Patency
Inspection	8/10
Lymphography	8/10
Isotopes	8/10
Histology	10/10

2.2.4 Function of Grafts

Function was measured by injecting isotopes (131 I gamma globulin) at the paw and measuring the activity at the groin region. A rise in activity similar to the contralateral side demonstrated function of the grafts (Fig. 2.34).

In untreated animals shortly after the injection at the paw, a rise in activity was measured at the groin. During the edematous phase, after the interruption of lymphatic flow, no activity was seen at the groin after injection. Following the reconstruction by lymphatic vascular grafts, a rise in activity was equivalent in comparison to normal untreated animals (Fig. 2.35).

Measuring the pressure within the lymphatic system peripheral to the side of grafting is another way to demonstrate the function of the grafts. A Statham element was used for this purpose. The zero point was at the level of the intralymphatic cannula.

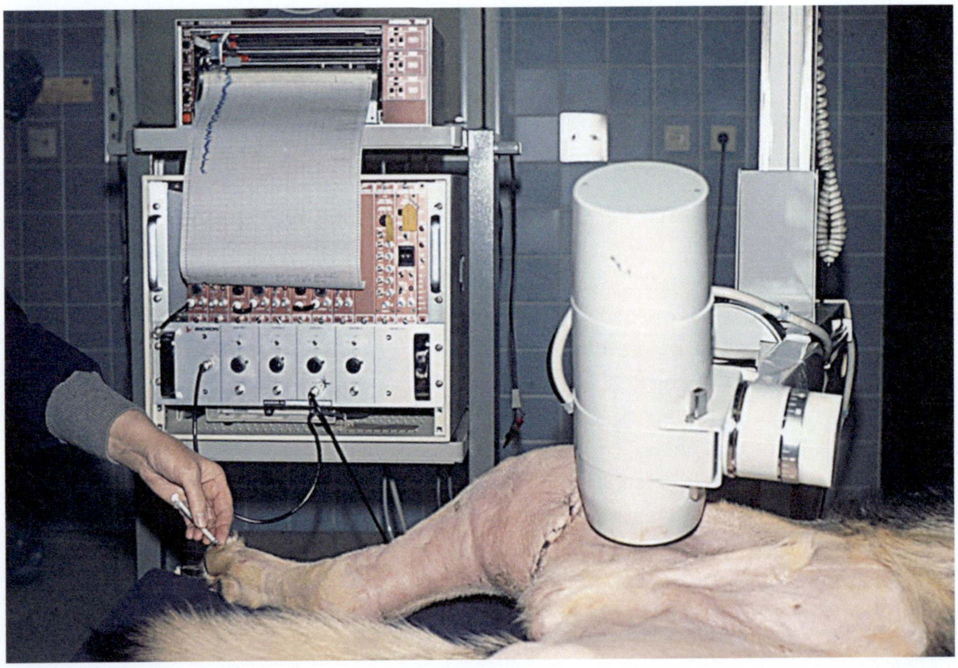

Fig. 2.34 Examination of function of lymphatic vessels grafts by isotopes injected at the paw and measured at the groin

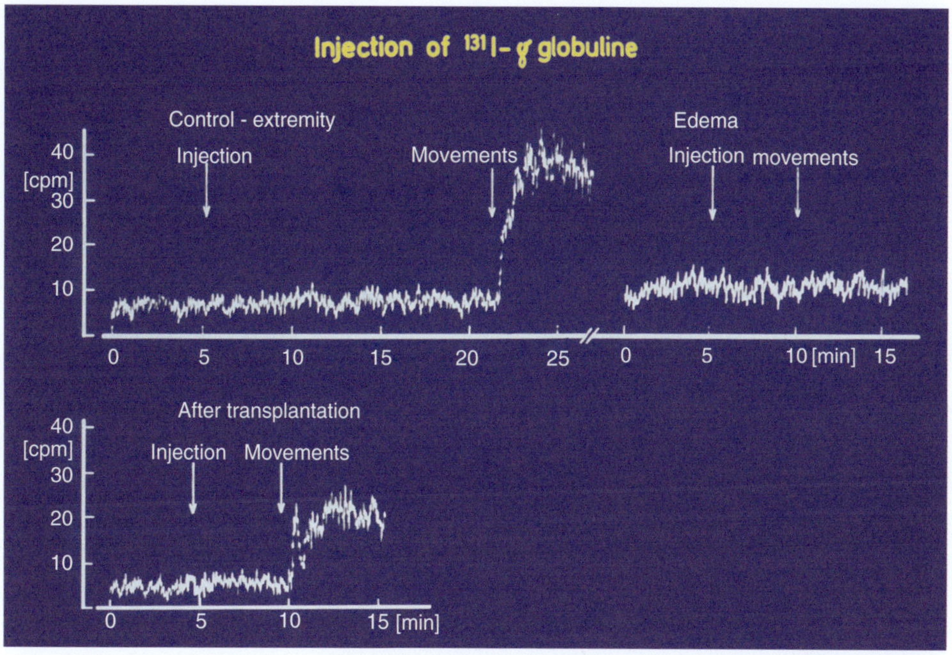

Fig. 2.35 Activity at the groin after injection at the paw in the contralateral control extremity, during the edematous phase and after reconstruction in the affected extremity (With permission Baumeister et al. 1981c, from Springer)

At the paw, in normal anesthetized dogs, the intra-lymphatic end pressure was 2.5 Torr. During edema the pressure was elevated significantly to 12.5 Torr. After transplantation of lymphatic vessels, the mean pressure of 3.5 Torr was found within the control range (Fig. 2.36).

The function was proved too by the measurements of the circumferences of the limbs at the paw, the metatarsus, and the lower leg as demonstrated in Fig. 2.30.

2.2.5 Investigations Using Different Materials for Extended Lymphatic Grafts

The conditions in a dog model are more similar to the human lymphedema than in the rat model. Especially longer grafts can then be used.

Segments of lymphatic collectors in the medial epi-fascial lymphatic system at the thigh were resected, and grafts with a length of about 6 cm were implanted using a tension-free anastomosing technique (Saumweber et al. 1988; Saumweber 1989).

Autologous and allogeneic lymphatic grafts, autologous venous grafts, and expanded PTFE prostheses with an inner diameter of 0.5 mm were used to reconstruct the interrupted lymphatic vessels.

The patency of the grafts was established by direct visual exploration and by dye injection. The ultrastructure of the transplanted vessels was studied using light, scanning, and transmission electron microscopy.

The observation period was 7–119 days.

All 14 autologous transplanted lymphatic vessels were patent during an observation period between 7 and 119 days.

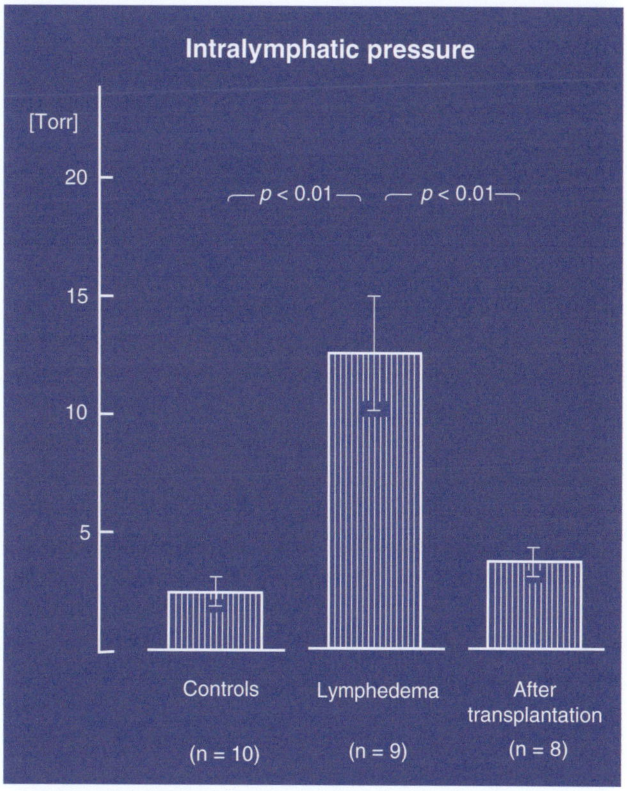

Fig. 2.36 Intra-lymphatic peripheral pressure, measured at the paw in controls, during the edematous phase and after reconstruction (With permission Baumeister et al. 1981c, from Springer)

No alteration during the whole observation period was seen at the histological examination of the autologous transplanted collectors.

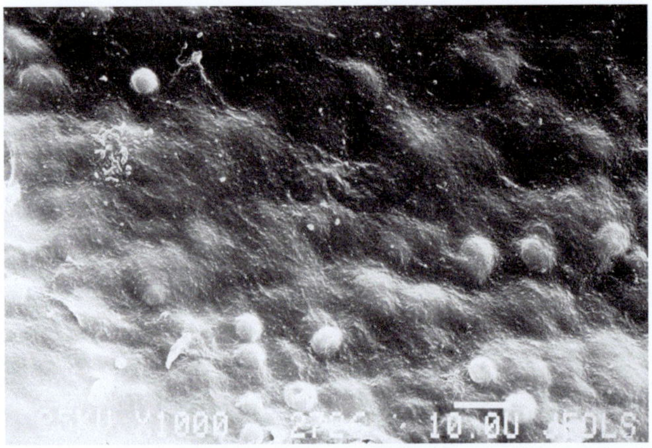

Fig 2.37 Intact epithelial layer in an autologous lymphatic transplant, 10 days after grafting (scanning electron microscopy, 1000-fold magnification)

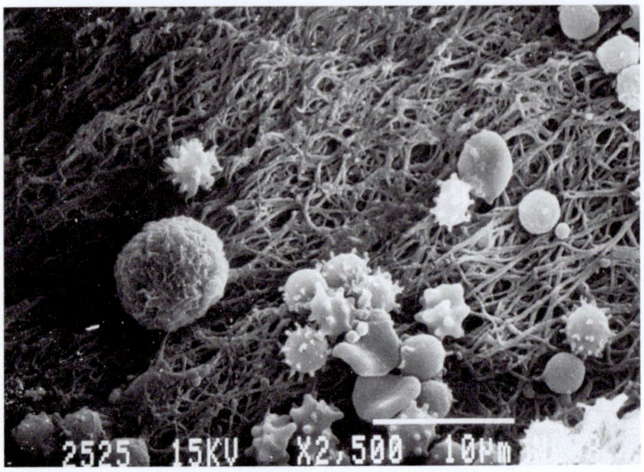

Fig 2.38 Inner surface of an allogeneic lymphatic transplant without endothelial surface, 21 days after surgery (scanning electron microscopy 2500-fold magnification)

Light- and electron microscopy revealed uniform and complete endothelial layer with prominent nuclei above elastic fibers in longitudinal direction. In the deeper sections of the wall, collagen fibers and smooth muscle cells were found. Figure 2.37 shows in the scanning electron microscopy a complete endothelial layer with prominent nuclei of the endothelial cells. Some erythrocytes are visible on top of the endothelial sheet.

Grafts in the allogeneic group ($n=14$) were patent only until the 21st day after transplantation. The grafting was performed without any immunosuppression. In the mongrel dogs, DLA typing has been performed beforehand. The host-recipient combination was proved different in two DLA loci.

In contrast to the autologous grafts, the endothelial cells of all allogeneic grafts began to form marked clouds. The intercellular junctions were separated, the endothelial layer breaking, and the deeper sections of the wall showed signs of disintegration. The endothelial cells have completely disappeared at day 21 after grafting. Later examinations did not show a re-endothelialization. The function of the grafts got lost. Figure 2.38 shows the inner aspect of an allogeneic lymphatic graft, 21 days after implanting. The former intima is severed. A pseudointima is built out of a fibrin net. On top one big monocyte, several lymphocytes and altered erythrocytes are seen.

A patency of about 70 % was seen replacing the lymphatics by small veins ($n=10$).

Pathologic changes like an intima proliferation were seen in venous grafts in various extensions shortly after the implantation. Within the same vessel, segments with and without proliferation were found. At the anastomosing site, the proliferation was especially prominent; however signs of recanalization were noticed in cases of obliterating proliferation (Fig. 2.39).

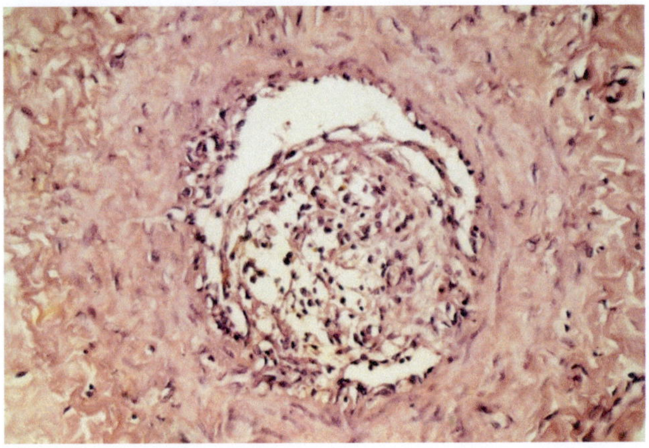

Fig. 2.39 Small venous transplant, partly occluded, 14 days after transplantation (H-E)

In the group of e-PTFE prostheses ($n=10$), all showed thrombosis already on day 7 after implantation (Fig. 2.40).

Histological investigations until day 45 showed a fibrin layer at the inner vessel wall, alterations by connective tissue ingrowth, and also sectors of normal texture of a neointima and a neo-adventitia (Saumweber et al. 1988; Saumweber 1989).

This comparative study showed us that autologous lymphatic vessel grafts are the best choice for a bypassing procedure as in reconstruction of a locally compromised lymphatic pathway.

Veins as grafting material replacing lymphatic grafts were also investigated by other groups

A comparison between lymphatic vessel grafts and vein grafts was performed by Yuwono and Klopper (1990). They also stated the advantage of lymphatic autografts in comparison to venous autografts.

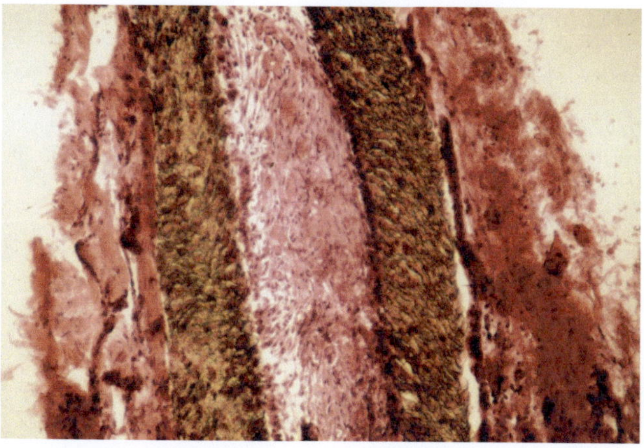

Fig. 2.40 Thrombosed and occluded PTFE implant 45 days after implantation

Thirty venous autografts were interposed at the dog's hind leg, bridging a lymphatic defect of about 6 cm. Ten of them were not irrigated before interposition, whereas 20 were irrigated with heparinized saline. Out of the 30 venous grafts, 26 were not found patent. All ten not irrigated vessels were occluded as well as 16 out of the 20 irrigated vessels. None was patent at and after an observation time of 2 weeks. Partially or total occlusion was found caused by a thrombus.

All autologous lymphatic grafts ($n=26$) with a length of 20 mm were patent during a reexploration 1–24 weeks after grafting.

The suture material (absorbable versus nonabsorbable) did not make a difference.

In none of the animals, a lymphedema did occur after harvesting (Yuwono and Klopper 1990).

Veins as grafting material for treating arm lymphedema in two patients were published by Holle and Mandel after experimental studies (Mandl 1981; Holle et al. 1982). In their previous experiments, they had found in 8 out of 12 dogs histologically patent grafts 6–12 weeks after interposition. They had used veins with a length of 10–15 mm. In all venous grafts, the wall was markedly fibrosed. Especially at the area of the anastomoses inflammatory infiltrates and granulations were observed.

Campisi and coworkers use venous grafts in cases where no lympho-venous anastomoses can be performed (Campisi 1991).

References

Baumeister RGH, Seifert J, Wiebecke B (1980) Transplantation of lymph vessels on rats as well as a first therapeutic application on the experimental lymphedema of the dog. Eur Surg Res 12(Suppl 2): 7–8

Baumeister RGH, Seifert J, Wiebecke B, Krumbach J (1981a) Lymph vessel transplantation for the treatment of experimental lymphedema in dogs. Eur Surg Res 13:40–41

Baumeister RGH, Seifert J, Wiebecke B (1981b) Homologous and autologous experimental lymph vessel transplantation: initial experience. Int J Microsurg 3:19–24

Baumeister RGH, Seifert J, Wiebecke B, Hahn D (1981c) Experimental basis and first application of clinical lymph vessel transplantation of secondary lymphedema. World J Surg 5:401–407

Baumeister RGH, Seifert J, Wiebecke B (1982a) Untersuchungen zum Verhalten von resorbierbarem und nichtresorbierbarem Nahtmaterial bei der Lymphgefäßnaht. Handchir Plast Chir 14:87–91

Baumeister RGH, Seifert J, Gabka C, Liebich H (1982b) Immunologisches Verhalten homolog transplantierter Lymphgefäße Immunologic Behaviour of Homologous Transplants of Lymphatic Vessels. Langenbecks Arch Chir Suppl Chir Forum 1982:37–41

Baumeister RGH, Goldmann U, Liebich H, Seifert J (1983) Ultrastrukturelle Untersuchungen zum Lagerungsverhalten von Lymphgefäßtransplantaten Ultrastructural Investigations of the Behaviour of Stored Lymph-Vessel Transplants. Langenbecks Arch Chir Suppl Chir Forum 1983:287–271

Campisi C (1991) Microchirurgia Applicata. Utet, Torrino

Clodius L (1977) The experimental basis for the surgical treatment of lymphedema. In: Clodius L (ed) Lymphedema. Thieme, Stuttgart, pp 44–78

Clodius L, Wirth W (1974) A new experimental model for chronic lymphedema of the extremities. Chir Plastic (Berl) 2:115–132

Cobbett J (1967) Small vessel anastomoses. Brit J Surg 20:16–20

Gabka JC (1983) Untersuchungen zur allogenen Transplantation von Lymphgefäßen bei Inzuchtratten. Promotionsschrift LMU, Muenchen

Goldmann U (1987) Untersuchungen zum Lagerungsverhalten von Lymphgefäßen. Inauguraldissertation, LMU Muenchen

Holle J, Mandl H, Kepler R (1982) Überbrückung eines Lymphgefäßdefektes mittels Veneninterposition (Eine experimentelle Studie). Handchir Mikrochir Plast Chir 14:83–86

Kressel M (1995) Primäre Rekonstruktion des Lymphabflusses bei der Dünndarmtransplantation an der Ratte. Promotionsschrift LMU, Muenchen

Mandl H (1981) Experimentelle Untersuchungen zur mikrochirurgischen Rekonstruktion von Lymphgefäßdefekten. Plastische Chirurgie 5:70–92

Saumweber DM (1989) Tierexperimentelle Untersuchungen zur Rekonstruktion von Lymphgefäßdefekten. Promotionsschrift LMU, Muenchen

Saumweber DM, Baumeister RGH, Liebich HG, Hammer C (1987) Untersuchungen zum Ersatz von Lymphgefäßen durch PTFE-Microgefäßprothesen Examination of PTFE Micro Vessel Prostheses Implanted within the Lymphatic System. Langenbecks Arch Chir Suppl Chir Forum 1987:191–194

Saumweber DM, Baumeister RGH, Liebich HG, Hammer C (1988) Experiences in experimental reconstructive microsurgery of lymphatics. In: Partsch H (ed) Progress in lymphology-XI. Elsevier Science Publishers B.V. (Biomedical Division), Amsterdam, pp 415–418

Sepulveda S, Baumeister RGH, Brooks W, Szymula von Richter TP, Hatz R, Lorenz B (1994) Investigations on resorption of long-chained fatty acids in small bowel transplantation with primary microsurgical lymphatic reconstruction. Lymphology 27(Suppl):861–863

Szymula von Richter TP, Baumeister RGH (1998) Clinical observation of intestinal transplantation with microsurgical lymphatic vessel and nerv reconstruction in the allogenic orthotopic rat model. Transplant Proc 30:2607–2608

Wallmichrath J, Baumeister RG, Deglmann CJ, Greiner A, Heim S, Frick A (2009) Technique and proof of patency of microsurgical lympho-lymphonodular anastomoses: a study in the rat model. Microsurgery 29:303–309

Wallmichrath J, Frick A, Baumeister RGH (2011) Microsurgical technique and function of lympho-lymphonodular anastomoses in the rat model. Lymphology 45(Suppl):343–346

Wallmichrath J, Baumeister RGH, Herrler T, Greiner A, Pieske O, Giunta RE, Frick A (2012) Experimental study on the microsurgical or spontaneous formation of lympho-lymphonodular anastomoses in the rat model. JPRAS 65:494–500

Wood RFM, Ingham Clark C (1991) Small bowel transplantation: future prospects. Immunol Lett 29:157–160

Yoffey JM, Courtice FC (1970) Lymphatics, lymph and the lymphomyeloid complex. Academic, London

Yuwono HS, Klopper PJ (1990) Comparison of lymphatic and venous interpositional autografts in experimental microsurgery of the canine lymphatics. Plast Reconstr Surg 85:752–757

3 Indication and Technique of Reconstructive Lymph Vascular Surgery

3.1 Indication and Prerequisites

Circumscribed impairment of the lymphatic system is the main indication for lymphatic grafting. In most cases, such a blockage results from surgical interventions such as lymphadenectomies in the axilla, groin, or pelvic area. Also dissections of lymphatic trunks in narrow parts of the lymphatic system, e.g., on the medial aspect of the knee, may lead to a lymphatic obstruction. In addition, infection or radiotherapy often damages the lymphatic pathways additionally and leads to the clinical manifestation of lymphedema.

A further indication exists for special forms of primary lymphedema with a regionally compromised lymphatic pathway, e.g., a unilateral lymphatic atresia at the groin and pelvis (Kinmonth 1982).

The following requirements have to be fulfilled prior to surgical treatment of secondary lymphedema (Table 3.1):

It is recommended to keep an interval of at least 6 months after the surgery or intervention, which has been followed by transitory swelling due to the interference with the lymphatic system. During that period of time, spontaneous normalization might occur, and lymphatic grafting may become superfluous. This time period should be used by complete decongestive therapy (CDT) which consists of manual lymph drainage, compression therapy, and exercises combined with skin protection.

After tumor therapy, an exact evaluation of the patient with respect to possible recurrence of the tumor is necessary.

In order to perform autologous lymphatic grafting, the harvest from the patient's thigh must be possible respecting residual lymphatic transport capacity after removal of the graft.

A preoperative lymphoscintigraphy permits evaluation of the lymphatic transport capacity in the donor region. If lymphatic flow is impaired in the donor region or there is swelling in the same region, lymphatic vessels should not be harvested.

The most important prerequisite is however the microsurgeon. He should have an extensive practice in microsurgery. Normally this deals however with vessels of more than 2 mm in diameter. Dealing with structures of less than 0.3 mm needs a considerable additional effort and therefore additional training.

The understanding and knowledge of lymphology is another prerequisite in order to avoid to be only a worker in a highly demanding manual field. The investigation of the patient, the appropriate indication, and the knowledge of managing complications and further possible treatment options need a profound expertise in the field of lymphatic diseases.

3.2 Equipment

The most advanced available microsurgical equipment should be used in order to facilitate the microsurgical demanding surgery on lymphatic vessels.

The microsurgeon should take advantage from the possible support to allow him just to move his hands and to get support for his forearms and elbows. Sometimes also breathing may be disturbing. It is advisable not to stop it with exertion, but to incorporate such periods within the workflow and repeat them more often instead of pausing for a longer time (Fig. 3.1).

The operating microscope is critical. It should allow high magnification of up to about 40-fold.

Improvements might be seen with addition of near-infrared light source allowing indocyanine green investigations during the surgery. However the visibility of lymphatic vessels is limited to the superficial area of the subcutaneous tissue. Therefore, the main lymphatic collectors which are located above the deep fascia may not be detected.

In order to manipulate the delicate lymphatic vessels, the finest microsurgical instruments available should be used. The tips of the pincers should measure not more than 0.1 mm.

R.G.H. Baumeister, *Reconstructive Lymph Vascular Surgery*, DOI 10.1007/978-3-319-31647-5_3

Table 3.1 Indication and prerequisites for lymphatic grafting

1. Circumscribed interruption or impediment of lymphatic flow
2. Undisturbed lymphatic system at least in one leg for harvesting
3. Lymphatic channels with a lumen at both sides of diseased area
4. Free of recurrence of malignant diseases
5. Capable for general anesthesia
6. Microsurgeon, experienced in microsurgery and lymphology as well

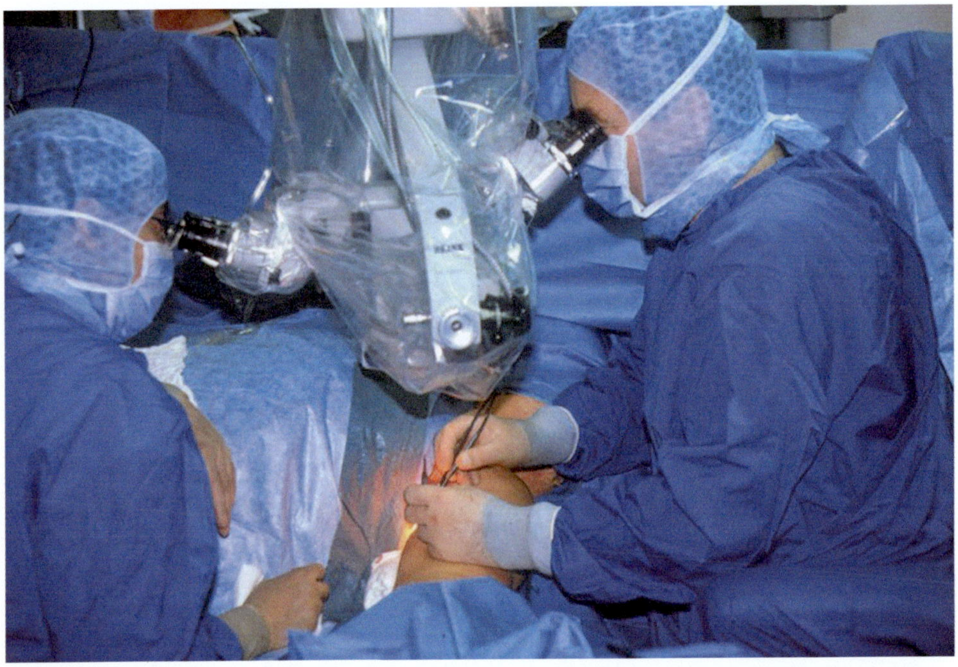

Fig. 3.1 Microsurgeon sitting in a chair with suspended forearms, operating microscope, ultrafine microinstruments

Also the suture material should be adapted to the size of the vessels to be anastomosed. In our personal experience in animals, we had the impression that reducing the foreign body reaction might be of advantage, looking at the histological findings showing large particles of the suture material next to the anastomoses. Since the production of polyglactin 910 (Vicryl®, Ethicon) with the size of 11-0 has been stopped, we use the remaining 10-0 (Baumeister et al. 1982).

However, nonabsorbable suture material, which is tinier than 12.0, might reduce the unfavorable correlation between vessel diameter and foreign body reaction.

Regarding the type of the needles, round needles are enough to penetrate the lymphatic vessel wall. For absorbable suture material, the smallest available needle size at the moment is BV 75-4.

To facilitate the suturing and handling the lymphatic vessels, a green plastic sheet is put underneath the vessels. Addition of some drops of Ringer's solution mixed with heparin helps to discriminate the front and back vessel walls by suspending the vessels.

3.3 Basic Technique

The basic technique follows the principles of vascular surgery and the adjustment to the special needs of lymphatic vessels. Elements were developed during the experimental phase of the reconstructive microsurgery of lymphatic vessels (Baumeister et al. 1981b, 1990, 2003).

3.3.1 Discriminating Lymphatic Vessels

Looking for lymphatic vessels is easy if they got stained. For staining, the dye has to get almost exclusively to the lymphatic system. This means that the molecular weight is relatively high in order to be ingested exclusively into the lymphatic capillaries. In Europe, Patent Blue V® is used for these purposes and fulfills these prerequisites (Fig. 3.2). The dye should be administered close to the subdermal lymphatic plexus. Thereafter it is quickly incorporated within the lymphatic system. Passive movements in anesthetized patients

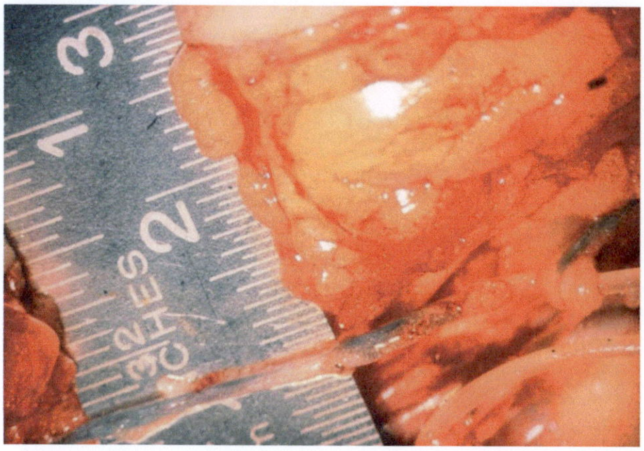

Fig. 3.2 Lymphatic collectors stained with Patent Blue V®

alleviate the transport to the base of the extremity within several minutes.

To search lymphatic vessels, a superficial incision just of the skin and dermis is recommended. By that way superficial tiny lymphatic vessels will not be harmed. Middle-sized lymphatic vessels in the subcutaneous tissue are located just within the adipose tissue or adjacent to major veins. The biggest lymphatic collectors are found mostly close to the deep fascia.

Underneath the fascia bigger lymphatic vessels can be found between the main arteries and veins.

Within the subcutaneous tissue, gently spreading movements in an oblique fashion to the main direction of the lymphatic vessels with a bigger instrument—I am using the "Metzenbaum" scissors—allow access to the stained lymphatic vessels. At the start of searching, one should try to get an overview of the vessels present in the corresponding area, e.g., the ventromedial bundle at the thigh. The surrounding tissue is separated from the lymphatic vessels. These are not touched until their course became obvious. Only prior to the harvest, the fine preparation starts. Intact bigger lymphatic collectors are relatively resistant against longitudinal tension. They can be elevated by fine hooks or also gently elevated by wet fingers.

In the edematous tissue, the lymphatic vessels do not get stained like in an undisturbed lymphatic flow. Therefore, we do not attempt to perform a staining like we do during the harvesting process. Therefore it is difficult to discriminate between small veins, small nerves, fibrous bands, and the altered lymphatic collectors. Since the area of search is limited and is performed in oblique direction, only a limited number of structures have to be checked.

The lymphatic collectors are mostly somewhat hidden within the subcutaneous tissue. The biggest ones are located just above the deep fascia. Lymphatic collectors are gray shining and are often separated from the surrounding adipose tissue. Small nerves instead have a bright white appearance and show oblique silver-shining stripes. The final decision sometimes can only be made after transection of the structure. Veins deliver blood. Out of the nerves prolapses the axon. A lymphatic collector should show a lumen without blood, preferentially delivering clear fluid.

In the treatment of a lymphocele, staining of the incoming lymphatic vessels is mostly possible. Blunt dissection of the distal part of the lymphocele directs to the incoming vessels. If fibrous tissue hinders the dissection from the outside, the lymphocele can be opened. The holes in the wall at the distal area, together with extrusion of stained fluid, will clarify the source of the lymphocele.

3.3.2 End-to-End Anastomosis

The two lymphatic vessels should be situated next to each other.

The first stitch is the most difficult one since the wall is collapsed. It might be helpful to add a small amount of Ringer's solution mixed with heparin helping to lift the wall (Fig. 3.3). In very small lymphatic vessels with fibrosis around the lumen, it might be advisable to only fix the outer layer with the stitches. The content of the lumen of the vessel can then drain into the graft.

The back wall is just lifted when starting to anastomose. The first stitch is placed at the far end of the vessels.

The sutures are directed from outside to inside and back on the opposite wall.

The second corner stitch is placed in front of the surgeon.

The suture is finished with the closure of the front wall.

Care should always be taken to avoid tension to the lymphatic vessel wall in oblique direction.

In longitudinal direction the vessel as a whole is however remarkable resistant against tension.

The number of stitches is dependent on the size of the lymphatic and the condition of the vessel wall.

Very small lymphatic vessels may just be adapted by one single stitch.

Danese (1982) had shown experimentally that lymphatic collectors may perform anastomosis by themselves if they come close to each other. This is encouraging for the microsurgeon. He will learn to minimize the disturbance for the lymphatic vessel.

In middle-sized lymphatic vessels, three to four stitches are enough.

Leakage will not be a problem since the pressure is low (Fig. 3.4).

In big or enlarged lymphatic vessels, around 6 to 8 stitches can be applied.

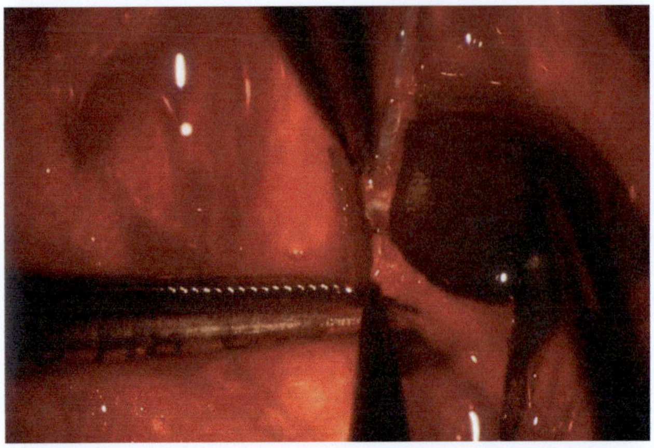

Fig. 3.3 End-to-end anastomosis, first corner stitch. Graft with translucent wall above, sclerosed lymphatic vessel of lymphedematous tissue with the lumen surrounded by fibrosed wall below (© Baumeister)

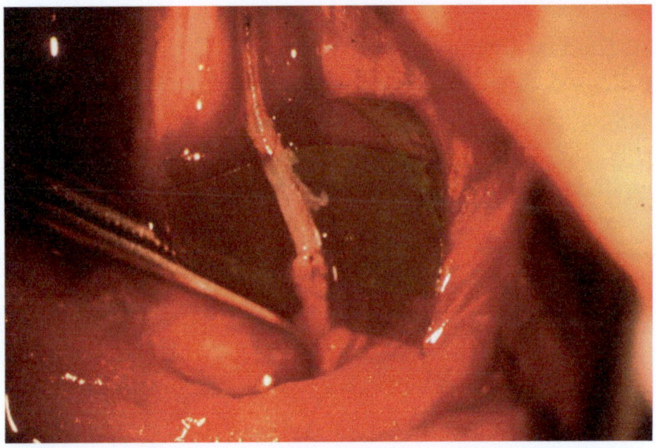

Fig. 3.4 End-to-end anastomosis completed. Graft filled with lymph (© Baumeister)

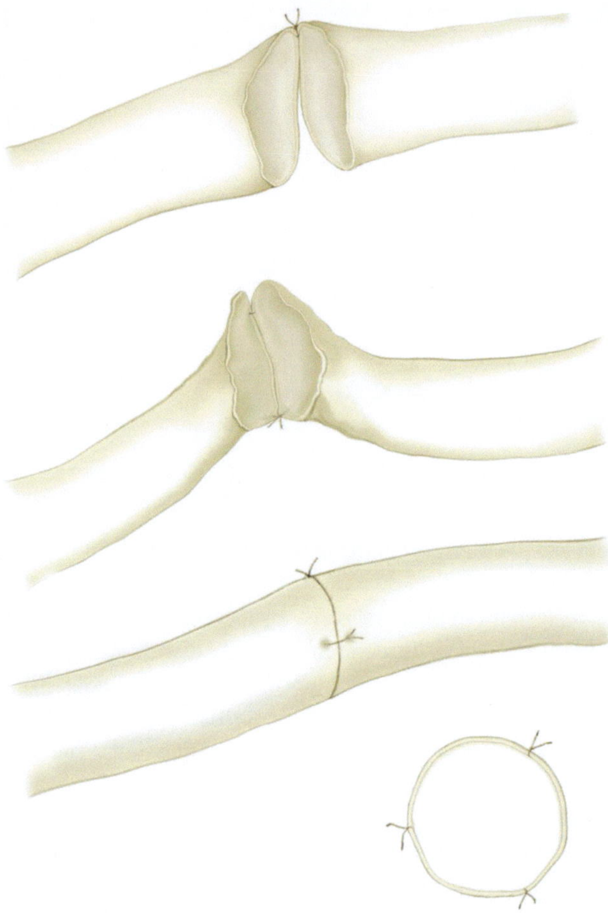

Fig. 3.5 End-to-end anastomosis with three stitches (© Baumeister)

The graft is filled with lymph at the end of the anastomosis also when the wall of the lymphatic vessel within the edematous tissue shows fibrosis (Fig. 3.5).

Different reason may contribute to this phenomenon.

A lumen can be seen also in lymphatic collectors in severe and long-standing lymphedemas.

Reconstruction within the lymphatic system does not need a pressure to work against another system like in lympho-venous anastomoses.

Lymphatic vessels are known for the active transport of the lymph. Lymphatic vessels continue pumping also in nutrient solution.

We saw recovery of activity along the lymphatic channels which was not present prior to the grafting in lymphedema patients in follow-up lymphoscintigraphies.

Therefore, a suction force produced by the lymphatic grafts can be postulated which helps to empty lymphatic vessels, also when they are not able to pump themselves.

The histological findings in lymphatic collectors, which have been chosen for anastomosis, underline the usefulness to perform reconstructive lymphatic surgery also in long-standing lymphedemas (Frick et al. 1990, 1992).

The example of a 50-year-old patient, 10 years after mastectomy and subsequent lymphedema of the arm, is shown in Fig. 3.6. The lumen is somewhat enlarged; endothelial cells are prominent.

3.3.3 End-to-Side Anastomosis

End-to-side anastomoses may be advisable if a lymphatic channel should not be transected, either to spare the normal flux or to give additional influx into a graft.

An oval excision into the wall is created. The stitches start either at the lowest part or at a point opposite to the surgeon in order to get a full view to the anastomosis until the last stitch. Collapsing of the wall can also be a problem. Therefore it might be helpful to fix the wall with one stitch first and to open the wall thereafter just next to it.

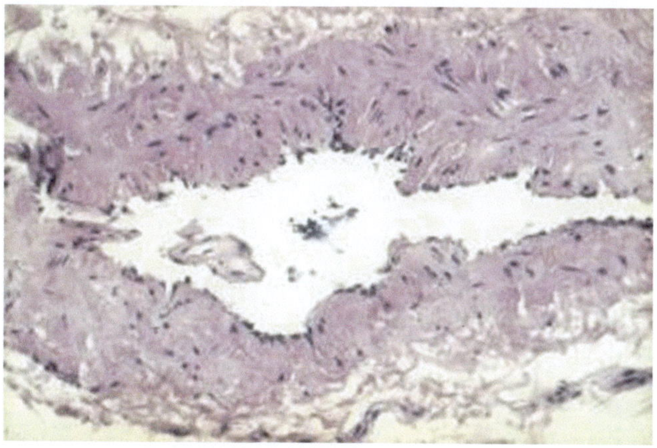

Fig. 3.6 Transection of an open lymphatic collector at the upper arm, selected for anastomosing, 10 years after mastectomy, somewhat distended lumen, prominent endothelial cell (H-E)

3.3.4 Harvesting of Grafts

At the thigh, there exists the ventromedial bundle which contains up to 16 lymphatic collectors (Kubik 1975, 1989). They spread out between the bottlenecks of the lymphatic system at the knee and the groin region. In between these two endangered regions, lymphatic vessels can be used for grafting. Even if one removes 2–3 vessels, more than three quarters of the vessels within the bundle remain untouched. Branches at the distal end allow additional anastomoses. Figure 3.7 shows two long free lymphatic grafts with branches at the distal end. The central endings are ligated. The threads have long endings which allow pulling at the grafts later on during the procedure.

Since often the grafts show also ramification prior to the entrance into the inguinal lymph nodes, also on both ends, additional anastomoses may be possible.

Staining of the vessel is important to facilitate the preparation and to identify functioning lymphatic vessels which will remain untouched. If however only two or three stained lymphatic vessels become visible, harvesting should not take place. For staining we use Patent Blue V ®. It is injected into the subdermis at the first and second web spaces. Passive movement of the joints leads to a quick transport toward the groin, which means that after about 15 min, the lymphatic vessels become stained with a blue-green color. Signs of dermal backflow, indicating deficiency in lymphatic transport, would be a contraindication for harvesting. For safety reasons, we perform a lymphoscintigraphy at the lower extremity in all patients who ask for lymphatic vessel transplantation, in order not to oversee an occult lymphatic transport problem.

The incision is started below the groin medial to the palpable femoral artery. We search for stained, bigger lymph collectors which are found above the deep fascia. We normally do not use stained lymphatic collectors adjacent to the greater saphenous vein since they are variable and not straight enough. From the starting point, we elongate the incision toward the knee, but we always stop above this area. Since the direction of the incision is adjacent to the direction of the lymphatic vessels, the incision is mostly somewhat curved toward the dorsal aspect of the thigh. The harvest is terminated proximal to the knee. Below that, connecting vessels are remained ensuring the undisturbed lymphatic flow (Fig. 3.8).

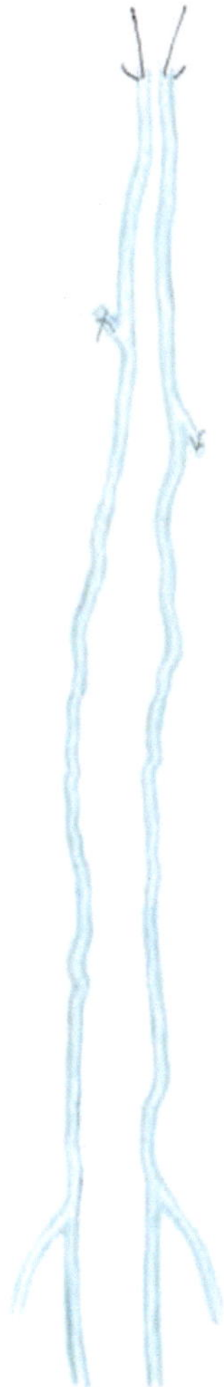

Fig. 3.7 Two lymphatic grafts with two additional peripheral branches, proximal ligatures with long threads to allow pulling (© Baumeister)

Since harvesting of lymphatic vessels is a crucial point, we recently also checked the lymphatic flow at the harvesting site performing lymphoscintigraphy. It was shown within a group of 19 consecutively investigated patients that there was an unchanged normal outflow after the harvest. The mean follow-up period was 4 years (Weiss et al. 2015).

In selected cases, where only moderate amounts of fat were present, we harvested the grafts in a minimally invasive way. We used two short incisions and dissected the

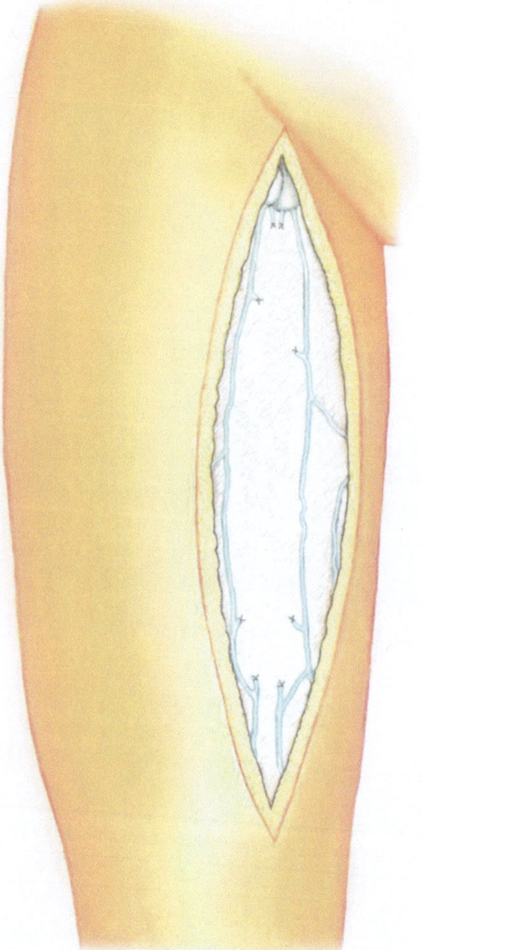

Fig. 3.8 Grafts have been harvested from the ventromedial bundle; peripheral connections to neighboring lymphatic vessels are remained (© Baumeister)

lymphatic vessels with the help of an endoscope. Through the endoscope the stained vessels could be seen clearly; however the overview about the bundle is limited (Baumeister et al. 2000).

3.3.5 Lymphatic Vessel to Lymph Node Anastomosis

Especially at the neck, it might be of advantage to connect the grafts directly to a lymph node.

Opening just the capsule of the node gives access to the marginal sinus. Bleeding should be avoided by careful preparation. The grafts are now adapted to the capsule with about four single stitches. Figure 3.9 shows a lymph node with two lymphatic grafts (above, one completely and one partly sutured) connected to the lymph node in the same way as two original lymphatic vessels (below, lateral).

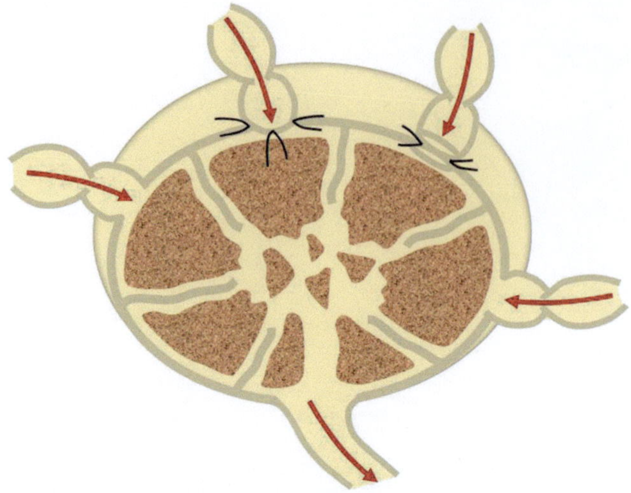

Fig. 3.9 Scheme of lymphatic vessel to lymph node anastomosis: two anastomoses, one partly finished (*right*), one completely finished (*left*) at the upper part of the node, connected to the marginal sinus like normal afferent lymphatic vessels (lateral on both sides)

3.4 Treating Edemas of the Upper Limbs

Most of edemas of the upper extremities are caused by an obstacle of the lymphatic system in the axillary region. In these cases this region has to be bypassed.

In all patients we perform a lymphoscintigraphy to verify the lymphatic transport deficiency.

In primary lymphedema, additionally an indirect lymphography, or nowadays a MRI lymphography, has to be performed since different defects besides a local interruption might be present and a treatment with lymphatic grafts therefore may not be advisable.

First, lymphatic collectors are searched below the axilla. Care has to be taken to keep away from irradiation fields. Depending on the length of the graft, the collectors are searched more distally to the axilla. Dependent also from the lymphoscintigraphic findings, collectors are searched more laterally, if the lymphedema is predominant in the draining area of the long cephalic pathway.

An oblique incision is performed transecting just the cutis. Underneath, the subcutaneous tissue is opened by blunt preparation. Since the biggest collectors are found just above the fascia, the searched is intensified there. Because in lymphedema a dye is transported mainly along the cutaneous lymphatic network and the transport is disturbed along the extremity, a dye is not applied at the edematous limb.

In order to facilitate the preparation and to save the lymphatic vessels, the search is performed under the microscope using a medium magnification.

In early stages of lymphedema, the lymphatic vessels have a gray, shiny appearance, and the lumen can be seen clearly after transection. As the lymphatic vessels undergo fibrosis in later stages of lymphedema, it becomes more difficult to discriminate between small nerves and fibrous cords. In this case, the final decision regarding their potential use for grafting can be made only after transection of the structure.

The nearest undamaged lymphatic system away from the upper arm is found at the neck region. The distance between the upper arm incision and the neck region is mostly equivalent or even less, compared to the length of the thigh and the distance between the groin region and the knee region. Lymphatic grafts can be used therefore in sufficient length.

The incision at the neck is performed about 2–3 cm above the clavicle at the dorsal border of the sternocleidomastoid muscle. It can be performed in one of the natural folds and will be hidden thereafter.

The sternocleidomastoid muscle is shifted medially or transected at the lateral border. Underneath, within the fat, lymphatic vessels and lymph nodes can be found.

The walls of the lymphatic vessels at the neck however are thinner than at the arms or the legs. Injection of dye subdermally behind the ear may facilitate the search for appropriate vessels. If the lymphatic vessels become stained appropriately, recognition is easy.

Suturing in this is area is often difficult because of the collapsing thin-walled vessels. Before transecting, it may be helpful to differentiate between the front and back walls by fixing the front wall with a suture.

A less demanding way exists in anastomosing the grafts with the lymph nodes. A superficial, oval incision is made in the capsule of the node, giving access to the marginal sinus. The graft is then connected with approximately four to six interrupted sutures.

To position the grafts between the two anastomosing sites, tubing from a drain is placed in the subcutaneous tissue between the incisions in the upper arm and the neck. Subsequently, the grafts are pulled through the wet drain gently and without friction. After removal of the tube, the grafts remain in the subcutaneous tissue free of tension. Care has to be taken that the grafts are pulled in the right direction according to the direction of the lymphatic flow (Figs. 3.10 and 3.11).

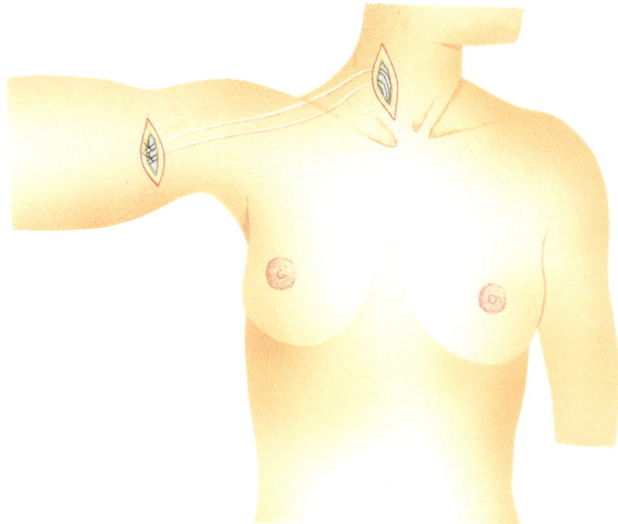

Fig. 3.10 Reconstruction of a lymphatic interruption in the axilla connecting lymphatic collectors at the upper arm and lymphatic vessels or lymph nodes at the neck by lymphatic autografts (© Baumeister)

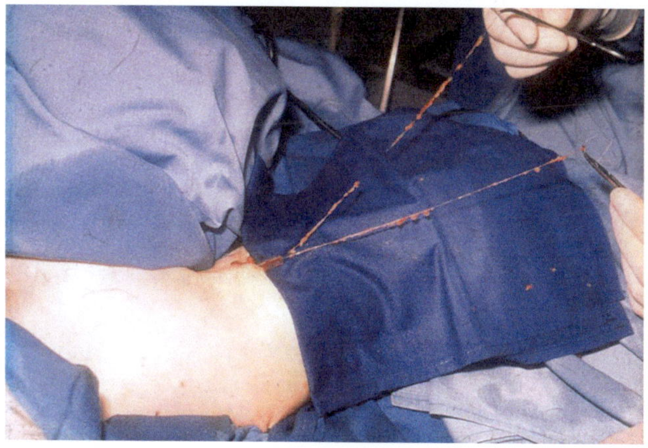

Fig. 3.11 Lymphatic vascular grafts ready for pulling them into a silicon tube which connects the incision at the upper arm with the incision at the neck (© Baumeister)

3.5 Treating Edemas of the Lower Limbs

Reconstruction of the lymphatic vascular system needs for harvesting one lower extremity which is not compromised at all regarding the lymphatic transport (Baumeister et al. 1981a). Additionally, an undisturbed lymphatic vascular system close to the area of obstruction should be present to take in the additional lymphatic fluid.

Treatment of edemas of lower limbs is therefore restricted to unilateral ones. The contralateral leg serves for harvesting. The undisturbed inguinal and pelvic lymphatic systems are then able to receive the lymph from the edematous side.

In all patients we perform a lymphoscintigraphy to verify the lymphatic transport deficiency.

In primary lymphedema, additionally an indirect lymphography, or nowadays a MRI lymphography, has to be performed since different defects besides a local interruption might be present and a treatment with lymphatic grafts therefore may not be advisable.

For unilateral edema of the lower limb, the grafts remain attached to the inguinal lymph nodes (Fig. 3.12). The endings of the grafts distally are closed with sutures with long endings. For transposing to the opposite side the grafts they are used for pulling.

Above the symphysis, a tunnel is created to connect the harvesting side and the area of anastomosing at the affected limb. A silicon tube is inserted temporarily to facilitate the transposing of the graft (Fig. 3.13).

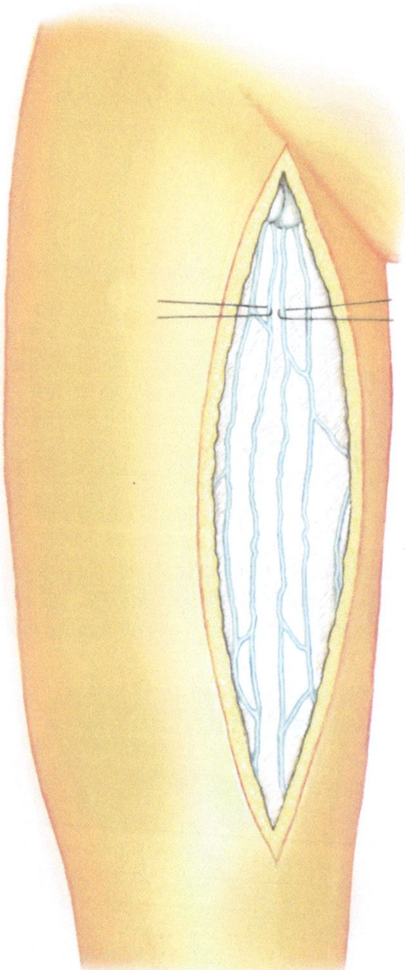

Fig. 3.12 Choosing two lymphatic collectors remaining attached at the lymph nodes for transposition in case of unilateral leg lymphedema (© Baumeister)

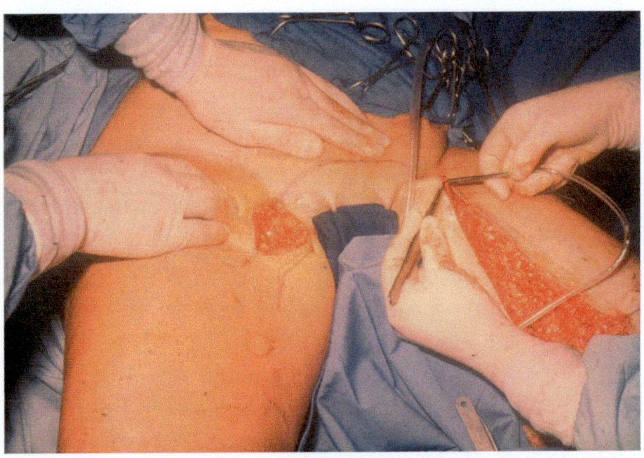

Fig. 3.13 Insertion of a tube between the incisions on the side of harvest and the affected limb for pulling the grafts without friction; tube is removed thereafter (© Baumeister)

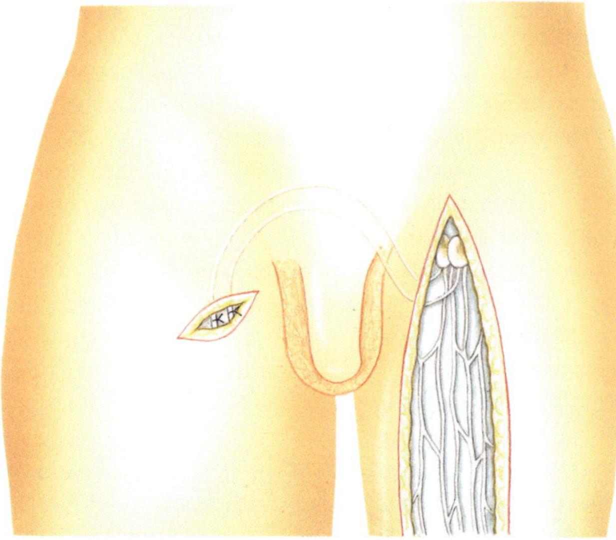

Fig. 3.14 Transposition of the grafts form healthy side to the affected limb, lymphatic anastomoses with ascending main lymphatic collectors (© Baumeister)

The distal ends of the grafts can easily be directed with prolonged threads of the suture. They get connected to one end of a bigger thread which has been inserted into the tubing of the drain before. The distal ends of the grafts are pulled into the tube and thus transposed to the opposite thigh. After removal of the tube and anastomosing the distal endings of the grafts with lymphatic vessels at the edematous side, the lymph flows in the correct direction. Lymph flows from the affected limb via the grafts to the lymph nodes of the healthy side. The lymph continues than the normal way, up to the thoracic duct and the left venous angulation (Fig. 3.14).

Exceptionally lymphatic grafting may also take place if both lower extremities are affected. This is the case when the area of obstruction is well defined and located at the distal part of the pelvis.

In one patient with resection of lymph nodes distally at the pelvis and proximally at the groin, lymphatic grafts have been harvested from the affected side and anastomosed to the distal inguinal lymph nodes and got attached to the central pelvic lymphatic tissue. By that way risk of additional swelling is restricted to the already edematous side. The patient improved clearly at the edematous side also at a follow-up period of more than 6 months.

3.6 Treating of Lymphoceles

Following surgical treatment, sometimes a lymphocele is remained, mostly located at the root of an extremity. This is a result of damage to the lymphatic vascular system. Transected lymphatic vessels fill the cystic structure. In cases with limited influx into the lymphocyst, they may be treated successfully by conservative means. Injection of small amounts of glucose with a concentration of 40–50% after emptying the lymphocele, followed by continuous slight compression, may induce gluing of the walls. If the overall lymphatic outflow of the limb however is persistently disturbed, the lymphocele may persist and lymphedema may occur. Especially in these cases, simple resection of the lymphocele and ligature of the lymphatic vessels which fill the lymphocele will not be sufficient. Reconstructive lymph vascular surgery has to search for the incoming vessels and connect them with grafts in these cases. By that way, the influx into the lymphocele is stopped, and the lymphocele may be resected with no risk of recurrency. Furthermore the graft can transport the arriving lymph into an undamaged lymphatic system which means that the reason for the edema is eliminated.

Examination prior to the surgery helps for an exact planning. Several methods are helpful.

With the onset of 3 T MRI lymphography, it became possible to show the exact entrance of the lymphatic vessels into the lymphocele (Notohamiprodjo et al. 2009).

With the combined help of lymphoscintigraphy and MRI lymphography, it is possible to show the connection between the way of lymphatic fluid and the filling of the cele (Notohamiprodjo et al. 2012).

Before starting the surgery, Patent Blue V ® should be injected subdermally at the periphery of the extremity. The incoming lymphatic vessels will become stained and can be identified and isolated (Fig. 3.15). If this does not work, the lymphocele should be opened and the entrances of vessels may be recognized from inside.

In cases showing a lymphocele close to the groin, lymphatic vessels can be transposed from the contralateral healthy side and drain the lymph to the healthy side (Fig. 3.16a, b).

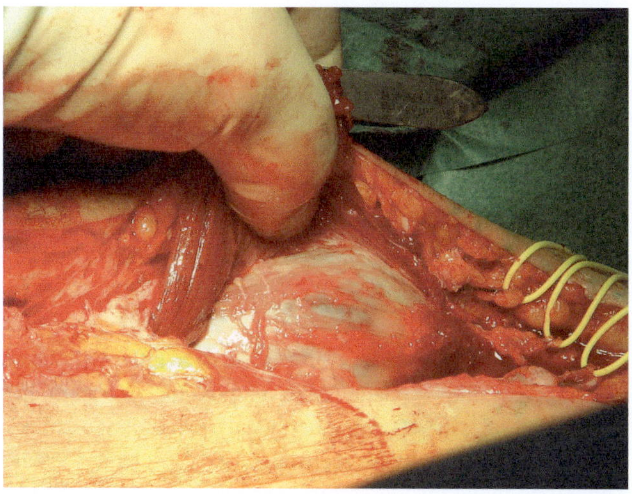

Fig. 3.15 Intraoperative view on the lymphocele and incoming stained lymphatic vessels, fixed with vessel loops (© Baumeister)

In lymphoceles close to the axilla, free lymphatic grafts taken from the thigh may connect the incoming lymphatic vessels to the healthy lymphatic system at the neck area like in cases suffering from lymphedema after axillary dissection.

If the use of a graft or transposing to undamaged lymphatic collectors nearby is impossible, lympho-venous anastomoses may be performed.

3.7 Treating of Lymphatic Fistulas

As one of a possible sequel of an injury to the lymphatic vessels, a lymphatic fistula may occur. This is the case when neighboring lymphatic vessels are not able to master the lymphatic load. The continuous elevated pressure leads to the persistence of the fistula. If with time the adjacent lymphatic vessels get adapted and are able to transport the lymphatic fluid, the fistula will dry up. Therefore first a conservative approach may be advisable.

If however the fistula persists, the feeding lymphatic collector should be identified first by MRI lymphography and lymphatic scintiscan (see also Fig. 5.29) (Notohamiprodjo et al 2009, Weiss et al. 2014) and finally during surgery with the help of intraoperative staining of the lymphatic vessels using Patent Blue V®. If possible, a reconstruction should be attempted, either by using a transposed lymphatic vessel from the opposite leg in case of a fistula close to the groin area (Fig. 3.17a, b), a free transplant for a fistula close to the axilla, or short free grafts in cases of a fistula in the periphery of an extremity. If reconstruction seems not to be possible, either a direct occlusion of the incoming lymphatic vessels or a deviation into an adjacent vein can be attempted.

3.8 Treating of Special Cases

Bottlenecks of the lymphatic system, like the medial aspect of the knee region or at the main lymphatic bundles at the lower leg, are endangered if surgical interventions or trauma interrupts lymphatic vessels to a greater extent.

This is a pattern of a localized blockade too. Lymphatic vessels in front and behind the interruption are in these cases able to bridge the gap (Fig. 3.18).

Edema of the penis and the scrotum may be also caused by a localized blockade of draining lymphatic vessels or lymph nodes, e.g., the medial ones at the groin. Under the condition of an undisturbed lymphatic outflow in at least one leg and open lymphatic vessels at the basis of the penis or scrotum, reconstruction is possible. Short lymphatic grafts terminating in the lateral inguinal lymph nodes are transposed to the penile and scrotal areas. There, anastomoses are performed with the lymphatics in the edematous area (Fig. 3.19).

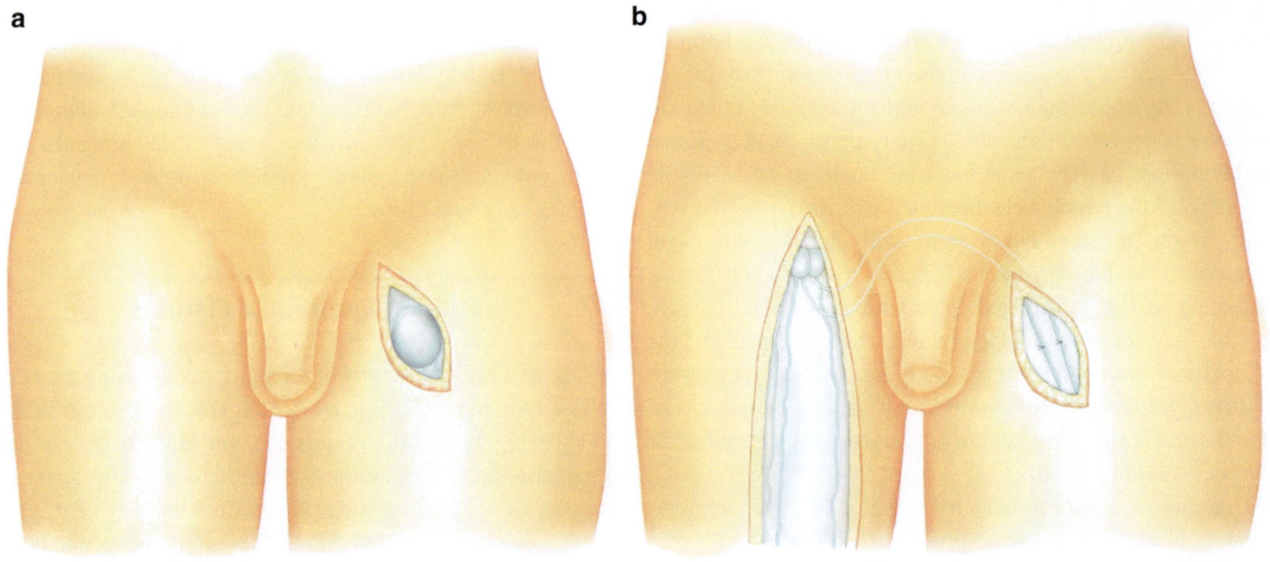

Fig. 3.16 (**a**) Lymphocele at the groin region filled by two incoming lymphatic collectors. (**b**) Lymphocele resected, incoming lymphatic collectors anastomosed to transposed lymphatic vessels from the healthy contralateral leg (© Baumeister)

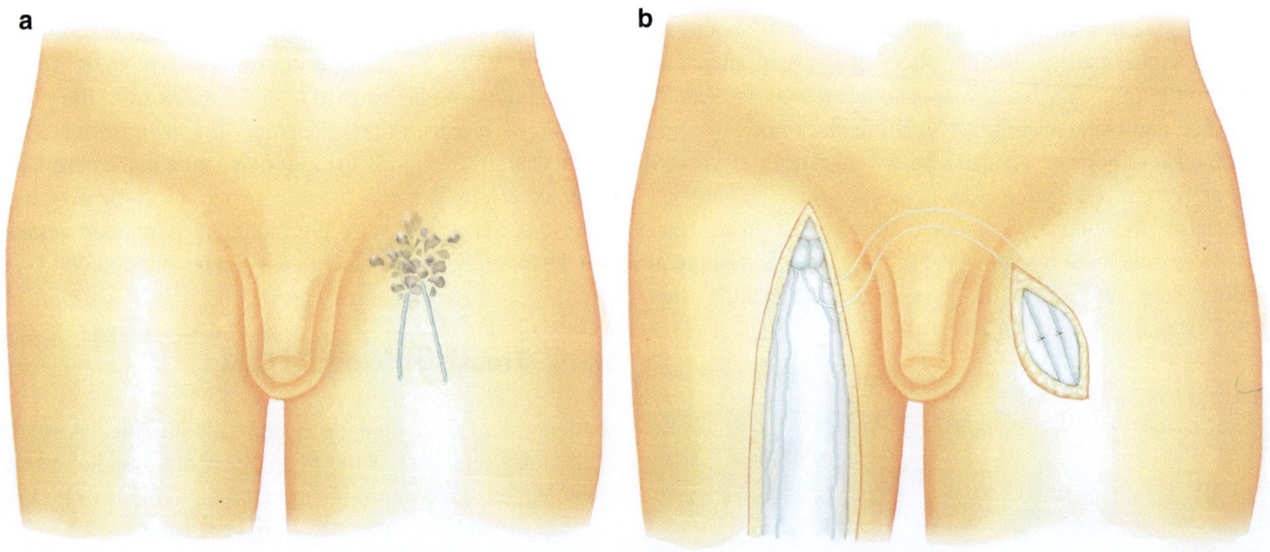

Fig. 3.17 (**a**) Lymphatic fistula at the groin with two open lymphatic collectors. (**b**) Lymphatic fistula resected two open lymphatic collectors anastomosed to two lymphatic vessels from the opposite leg (© Baumeister)

In primary lymphedemas too, localized atresia or agenesis of the lymphatic system may be the cause of lymphedema. Kinmonth (1982) described in his book: The Lymphatics a type of lymphedema which is due to a localized and unilateral atresia of the lymphatic system at the groin or the pelvic region. The distal lymphatic system was normal in the direct lymphography. In these special cases of primary lymphedemas also transposing of healthy lymphatic vessels from the opposite thigh is possible. Beneath the absent or diminished lymphatic nodes, the lymphatic collectors are anastomosed with the transposed lymphatic vessels. The lymph may flow thereafter to the contralateral lymphatic nodes and further on toward the pelvic chains at the not affected side like in unilateral secondary lymphedemas.

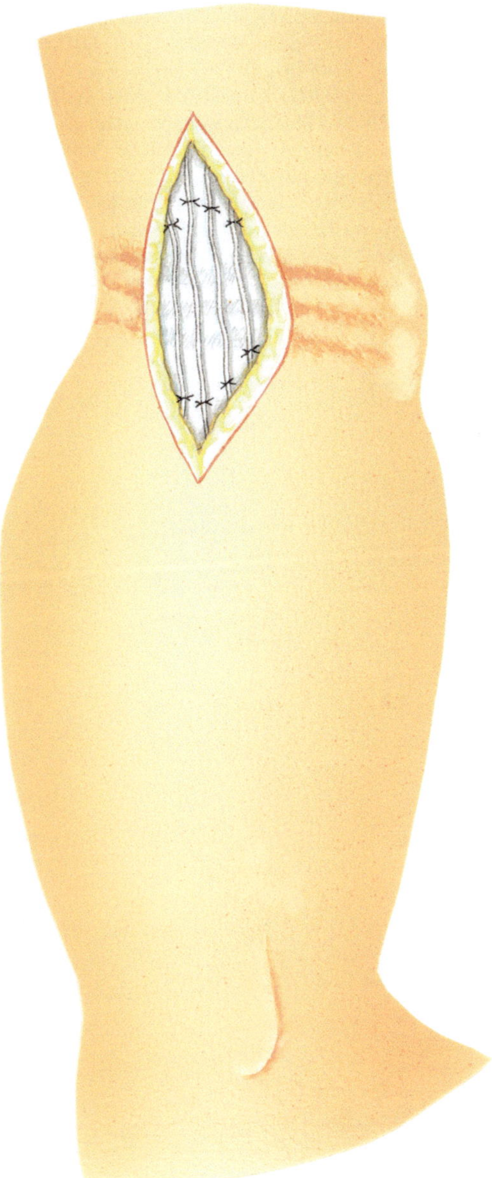

Fig. 3.18 Reconstruction of an interrupted lymphatic pathway at the knee (© Baumeister)

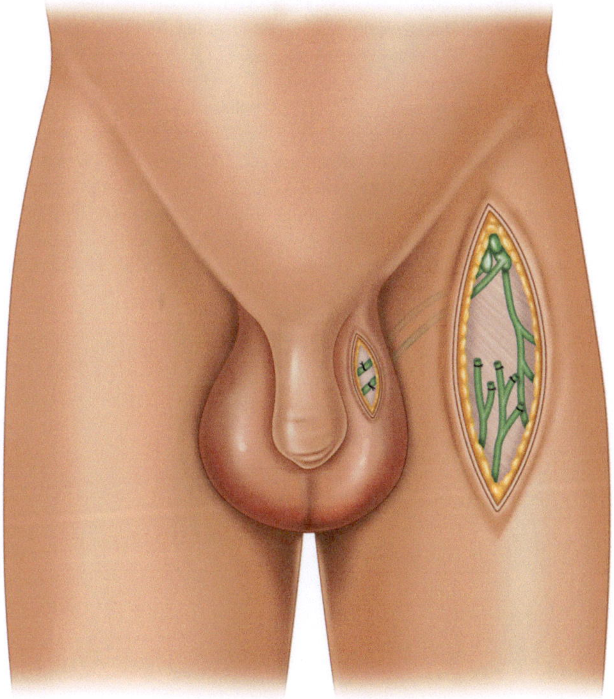

Fig. 3.19 Transposition of lymphatic grafts, connected to the lateral lymph nodes at the groin in penile and scrotal lymphedemas

References

Baumeister RGH, Frick A (2003) Die mikrochirurgische Lymphgefäßtransplantation. Handchir Mikrochir Plast Chir 35:202–209

Baumeister RGH, Siuda S (1990) Treatment of lymphedema by microsurgical lymphatic grafting: what is proved? Plastic Reconstr Surg 85:64–74

Baumeister RGH, Seifert J, Hahn D (1981a) Autotransplantation of lymphatic vessels. Lancet 17:147

Baumeister RGH, Seifert J, Wiebecke B, Hahn D (1981b) Experimental basis and first application of clinical lymph vessel transplantation of secondary lymphedema. World J Surg 5:401–407

Baumeister RGH, Seifert J, Wiebecke B (1982) Untersuchungen zum Verhalten von resorbierbarem und nichtresorbierbarem Nahtmaterial bei der Lymphgefäßnaht. Handchir Plast Chir 14:87–91

Baumeister RGH, Frick A, Krumbach J (2000) Microsurgery and endoscopy in the treatment of lymphatic blockades. Lymphology 33(Suppl):254–257

Danese C, Bower R, Howard J (1982) Experimental anastomosis of lymphatics. Arch Surg 84:24

Frick A, Wiebecke B, Baumeister RGH (1990) Histologische Befunde von Lymphgefäßen, gewonnen bei Lymphgefäßtransplantationen. In: Baumeister RGH (ed) Lymphologica Jahresband 1990. Medikon, Muenchen, pp 103–105

Frick A, Wiebecke B, Baumeister RGH (1992) Pathologisch-anatomische Veränderungen proximaler Lymphkollektoren bei Lymphödemen. In: Behrens v. Rautenfeld D, Weissleder H (eds), Lymphologica Jahresband 1992. Medikon, Muenchen, pp 68–70

Kinmonth JB (1982) The lymphatics. Edward Arnold, London

Kubik S (1975) Zur klinischen Anatomie des Lymphsystems. Verh Anat Ges 69:109

Kubik S (1989) Anatomie des Lymphgefäßsystems. In: Földi M, Kubik S (eds) Lehrbuch der Lymphologie. Gustav Fischer, Stuttgart, pp 1–184

Notohamiprodjo M, Baumeister RGH, Jakobs TF, Bauner K, Boehm H, Horng A, Reiser MF, Glaser C, Herrmann KA (2009) MR-lymphangiography at 3.OT- a feasibility study. Eur Radiol 19:2771–2778

Notohamiprodjo M, Weiss M, Baumeister RGH, Sommer WH, Helck A, Crispin A, Reiser MF, Herrmann KA (2012) MR Lymphangiography at 3.0.T: correlation with lymphoscintigraphy. Radiology 264:78–87

Weiss M, Burgard C, Baumeister R, Strobl F, Rominger A, Bartenstein P, Wallmichrath J, Frick A, Notohamiprodjo M (2014) Magnetic resonance imaging versus lymphoscintigraphy for the assessment of focal lymphatic transport disorders of the lower limb. Nuklearmedizin 53:190–196

Weiss M F, Baumeister RG, Zacherl MJ, Frick A, Bartenstein P, Rominger A (2015) "Mikrochirurgische autologe Lymphgefäß-Transplantation: Verursacht die Entnahme von Lymphgefäß-Transplantaten Lymphtransportstörungen an der Spenderextremität? (Microsurgical autologous lymph vessel transplantation: Does harvesting lymphatic vessel grafts induce lymphatic disturbances of the donor limb?) Handchir Mikrochir Plast Chir 47:359–364

4 Methods for Objectification of the Results

4.1 Volume Measurement

Changes after any kind of edema treatment in extremities should be measured as exactly as possible. Measurements of circumferences at single points reflect the differences insufficiently.

Measurement of volumes is more accurate.

We used the method according to Kuhnke (1976) which is widespread in Germany. The volume is calculated from measuring the circumferences at a distance of 4 cm. The measuring can be simply performed just with the help of a tape measure.

Kuhnke described different ways of calculating (Kuhnke 1976, 1978).

The disk model is the most appropriate one. The volume of the disk with a height of 4 cm is calculated having measured the circumference.

Circumference and volume are connected according to the equation:

$$U^2 = \frac{4\pi}{h} \times V$$

Since the height is 4, the equation is simplified:

$$\frac{U^2}{\pi} = V$$

The volumes of the disks are then added up and result in the volume of the extremity within the measured area (Fig. 4.1).

Different methods for calculating the volume have been described. They are comparable if used in the same way during the investigation.

The optoelectronic method calculates continuously the volume by measuring the diameter of the extremity in two directions, moving a frame over the extremity.

During the procedure of the water replacement method, the extremity is immersed into a tube filled with water, and the water which is driven out is measured.

These methods are basis of investigations from other groups.

4.2 Nuclear Medical Investigation

Another important way to follow the results of treatment is to assess the function of the lymphatic system.

In order to repeat the measurements, a low-invasive procedure is necessary.

For quantification different ways have been proposed. Determining and measuring regions of interest require a strict protocol to give reproducible results.

Therefore the Department of Nuclear Medicine at the LMU performed lymphoscintigraphies without determining regions of interest. It is stated that this is a low-invasive, versatile, simple technique, which may be suited well to assess lymphatic function.

Verbal description of lymphoscintigraphic findings alone however fails to evaluate the different findings.

Therefore visually five criteria were assessed and scored:

The lymphatic transport kinetics, *K*:

0, no delay
3, low-grade delay
5, extreme delay
9, missing transport

The distribution pattern, *D*:

0, normal distribution, i.e., nearly no background
3, partial diffuse (e.g., only in the surroundings of a knee)
5, diffuse distribution
9, transport stop

The time to appearance of lymph nodes, *T*:

Time in minutes to the first appearance of regional lymph nodes
9, no appearance

R.G.H. Baumeister, *Reconstructive Lymph Vascular Surgery*, DOI 10.1007/978-3-319-31647-5_4

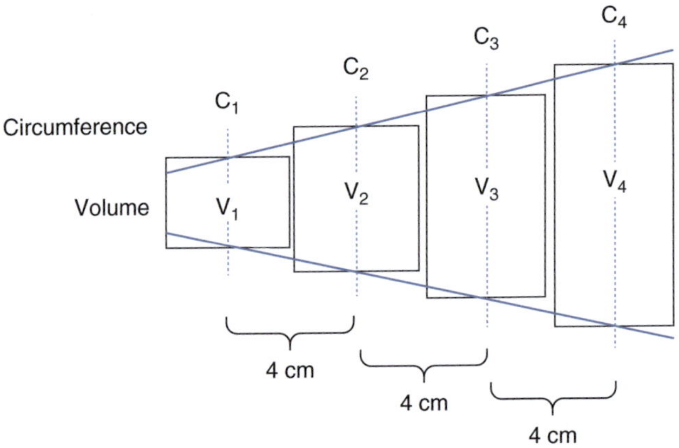

Fig. 4.1 Calculating the volume of an extremity by the disk model according to Kuhnke, adding the volumes of the disks with a height of 4 cm, measuring the circumference at the middle of single disks

The assessment of lymph nodes, *N*:

0, clearly demonstrated
3, faint visualization
5, hardly recognizable
9, no visualization

The assessment of lymphatic vessels, *V*:

0, clearly demonstrated
3, faint visualization
5, hardly recognizable
9, no visualization

"The transport index (TI) is then calculated by the formula

$$\mathrm{TI} = K + D + 0.04T + N + V$$

The rational for this formula is that all criteria are considered as equivalent.

Score values range from 0 to 9 including all integer numbers. Thus, TI values range between 0 (normal) and 45 (pathological) (Fig. 4.2, Table 4.1).

Normalization of *T* (min) is performed by the factor 0.04, i.e., 200 min (maximal delay of lymph node appearance) yields the score value 8. No appearance is evaluated by 9."

An interobserver study in 179 investigations was performed. A second observer reassessed the 179 limbs without knowledge of the results of the first observer. The mean difference for TI was rather small (2.61). The correlation was 0.96.

Using TI=10 to discriminate between normal and pathologic lymph drainage in 122 investigation, 38 were found true positive, 75 true negative, 8 false positive, and only 1 false negative. Thus, sensitivity was 97.4 % and specificity 90.3%.

Although evaluation of lymphatic transport kinetics depends on the experience of the investigator, a good reproducibility was demonstrated ($r=0.96$).

Therefore, that quantification of scintigraphic findings has proved very useful especially in follow-up studies. This method was used therefore to control the effect of reconstructive lymph vascular surgery in different studies (Kleinhans et al. 1985; Weiss et al. 2002, 2003).

All patients are investigated prior to surgery. At the lower extremity, the possibility of harvesting is clarified by lymphoscintigraphy, looking for a possible deficiency in lymphatic transport. At the edematous extremity, lymphoscintigraphy is performed in order to get an impression about the severity of the disturbance in lymphatic transport. Additionally it provides information about residual areas of less disturbed lymphatic outflow, and it serves as basic information for follow-up studies (Weiss et al. 2015a). About 1 year after surgery and for follow-up studies, lymphoscintigraphies are performed at the affected extremities. Figure 4.3 shows the example of a normal lymphoscintigraphy at the lower extremity. It was performed in order to check the possibility for harvesting a lymphatic graft.

In a recent study also the sequela of the harvest with respect of the lymphatic transport at the donor limb was investigated. In 19 consecutive patients 49 months after the harvest all values of the TI were close to the preoperative value and within the normal range. The results showed that microsurgical transfer of lymph vessel grafts is possible without compromising lymphatic drainage of the donor limb if safety precautions are taken into account (Weiss et al. 2015b).

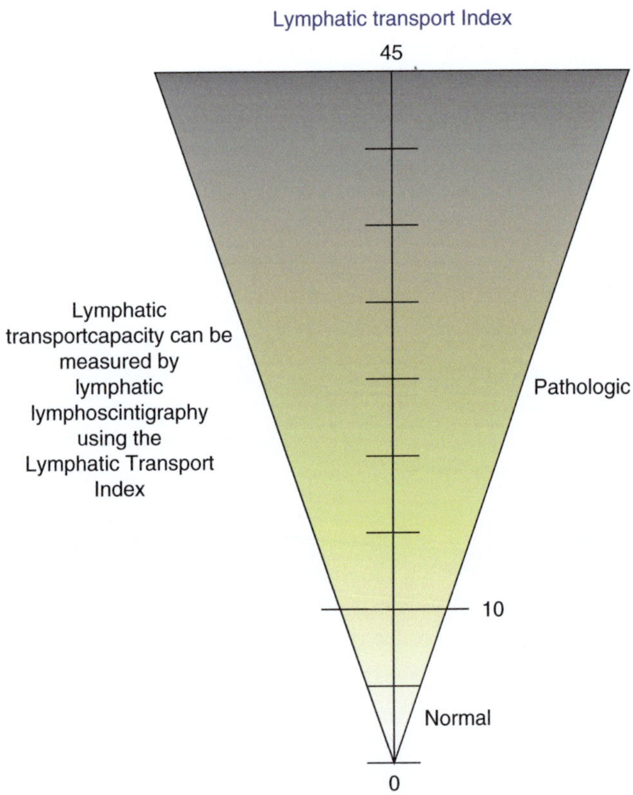

Fig. 4.2 Scheme of the lymphatic transport index

Table 4.1 Lymphatic transport index

Transport index					
	Kinetics	Distribution	Time	Lymph nodes	Lymphatic vessels
	K	*D*	*T*	*N*	*V*
0	No delay	Normal	$n = 0.04 \times$ minutes	Clearly demonstrated	Clearly demonstrated
3	Low-grade delay	Partial diffuse		Faint visualization	Faint visualization
6	Extreme delay	Diffuse		Hardly recognizable	Hardly recognizable
9	Missing transport	Transport stop	No appearance	No visualization	No visualization

Transport index (TI 0–45; pathologic ≥ 10)

4.3 Indirect Lymphography

To prove the patency of lymphatic grafts by direct visualization is difficult.

Oily contrast medium was a long time used agent. However it harms the lymphatic vessels. In our experiments we found lymphatic anastomoses occluded after contact with the contrast medium. Furthermore, it would be necessary to sacrifice a lymphatic vessel in order to perform the injection.

Water-soluble contrast medium is another possibility to show lymphatic vessels. The contrast medium should be administered subepidermally at an average infusion rate of 0.12 ml/min with the aid of thin butterfly needles (size 20–25) and an infusion pump. Exact subepidermal positioning of the tip of the needle is of paramount importance to facilitate a "contrast depot" from which lymphatics fill (Partsch et al. 1988).

According to our experience, lymphatic vessels are shown normally in a distance of several centimeters. Occasionally however the dye finds its way to more distant located bigger vessels. In these cases also the grafts can be visualized.

The example in Fig. 4.4 shows a lymphatic graft above the clavicle 4 years after bypassing the axilla. Visualization was possible with the help of indirect lymphography using water-soluble contrast medium (Isovist®).

4.4 MRI Lymphangiography

Vascular surgery needs urgently a method to visualize the vessels. Advancements are necessary in order to visualize the tiny lymphatic vessels not only superficial beneath the skin like indocyanine green method or at short distances like the indirect lymphography. MR lymphangiography is a promising method to visualize the lymphatic without such restrictions. Contributions for further development have been made by the Institute for Clinical Research at the LMU. Since the method is elaborated, only in selected patients MRI lymphangiography has been used to prove patency and to clarify the lymphatic system preoperatively.

"MR-lymphangiography (MRL) with extracellular gadolinium derivatives has been shown by Lohrmann et al. (2006) to be a safe and feasible investigation for primary and secondary lymphedema, providing valuable anatomical information with high spatial and temporal resolution.

With MRL, the entire lower extremity can be examined in several steps. Fat-saturation techniques render image

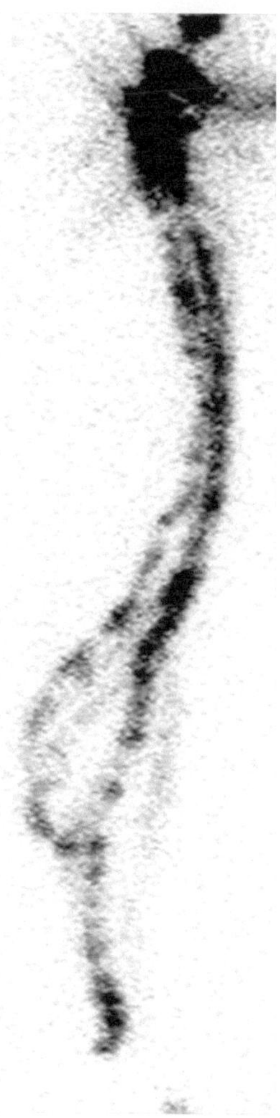

Fig. 4.3 Example of a normal lymphoscintigraphy at the lower extremity, checking the possibility for harvesting a lymphatic graft

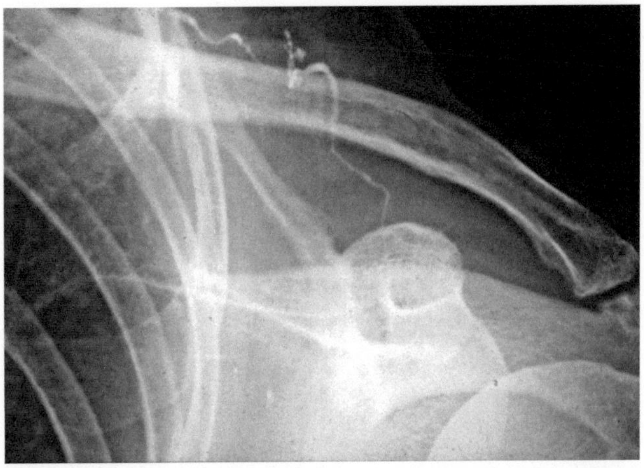

Fig. 4.4 Indirect lymphography using water-soluble contrast medium (Isovist®) showing a lymphatic graft above the clavicle 4 years after bypassing the axilla (© Baumeister)

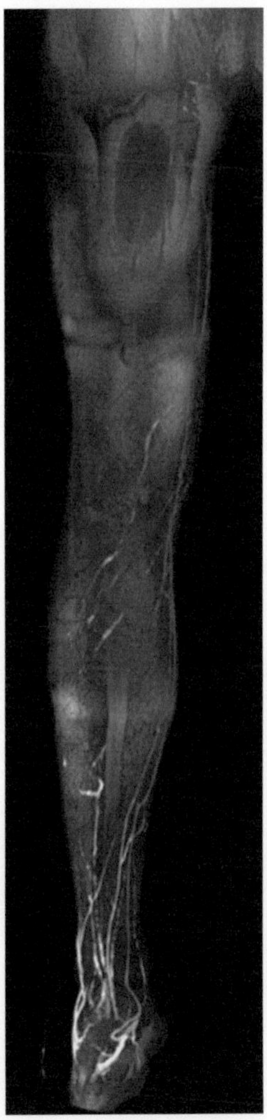

Fig. 4.5 Example of a normal MRI lymphography of a lower extremity

subtraction dispensable and allow for time-efficient acquisition (Lohrmann et al. 2007).

However, in plane resolution of MRL is limited at 1.5 Tesla (1,2,x1,2x1,1 mm^3) following constraints associated with the field strength (Lohrmann et al. 2008), so that the depiction of typically delicate lymph vessels, with sub-millimeter diameters, may be difficult (Lohrmann et al. 2006).

The introduction of higher field strength at 3.0 Tesla and multichannel coils provide a higher signal gain, which can be invested in high spatial resolution and isotropy to generate 3D data sets with options for 3D postprocessing (Michaely et al. 2007).

Furthermore, parallel imaging techniques reduce acquisition time with negligible signal penalty (Schoenberg et al. 2005). This high-resolution depiction of lymph vessels may help to enhance the understanding of anatomical and morphological details and to identify potential donor vessels for lymph-vessel transplantation, information that is crucial in selected patients when physiotherapy is not effective enough (Baumeister et al. 1981)."

The introductory remarks by Notohamiprodjo et al. (2009) for a feasibility study regarding MR lymphangiography at 3.0 T describe the development of MR lymphangiography very well.

After injection of gadolinium, lymphatic vessels are visualized along the extremity. For lymph vascular surgery, it is important that also the main collectors which run above the fascia are visualized. Figure 4.5 shows an example of a normal MRI lymphography of the lower extremity.

Since the potential of MRL at 3.0 Tesla with parallel imaging techniques and ultrahigh spatial resolution was unknown, a prospective study was performed to establish an imaging protocol for contrast-enhanced MRL of the lower extremity to investigate the value of this technique to visualize peripheral lymphatic vessels and to describe the MR morphology of normal and abnormal lymphatic vessels in extremity lymphedema (Notohamiprodjo et al 2009).

This is of special interest for the investigation in primary lymphedema since the knowledge of the status of lymphatic vessels is crucial to clarify the possibility for lymphatic vessel transplantation.

Sixteen patients were examined with a highly resolved isotropic T1w-3D-GRE-(FLASH) sequence (TR 3.76 ms/TE 1.45 ms/FA 30°/voxel size 0.8×0.8×0.8 mm^3) at 3 Tesla MRI after intracutaneous injection of gadolinium-diethylenetriamine-pentaacetic acid.

Two radiologists evaluated overall image quality, contrast between the lymphatic vessels and background tissue, venous contamination, visualized levels, and fat saturation homogeneity on 3D maximum intensity projections.

Overall image quality was good to excellent, and all examinations were diagnostic except one, where contrast medium was injected subcutaneously instead of intracutaneously.

Overall image quality was good to excellent in 12/16 cases. Depiction of lymphatic vessels was good to excellent in 15/16 cases. Venous contamination was always present, but diagnostically problematical in only one case.

Instant lymph drainage was observed in unaffected extremities, reaching the pelvic level after approximately 10 min.

Lymph drainage was considerably delayed in lymphedematous extremities. Ectatic lymphatic vessels, entrapment, and diffuse drainage of contrast medium correlated with impaired lymph drainage.

Based on these findings, MRL became a valuable tool for microsurgical treatment planning especially in primary lymphedemas and in patients with lymphatic fistulas and lymphoceles.

Also monitoring in selected cases with and without comparing to the functional findings in lymphoscintigraphy was successfully performed (Notohamiprodjo et al. 2012).

4.5 Quality of Life Assessment

In evidence-based medicine, studies are generally based on objectivity, and treatment outcomes are assessed by their effects. Particularly for chronic and malignant diseases, which impair patient's everyday life, it is necessary to apply additional and new criteria to judge the outcomes. Outcomes of medical treatment assessed traditionally by parameters like "death rate" or "survival rate" are now evolving to not only "whether" or "for how long" there is a possibility of survival but "how is the life worth living" and "how harmful" is the situation which may be the most important points of view particularly from the patient's perspective (Koller and Kussmann 1995).

To assess general health and whether lymphatic vessel transplantation was a successful treatment from the patient's point of view, we developed a specially designed questionnaire (Springer 2011; Springer et al. 2012). We started with the standardized SF-12 quality of life instrument. This is a shortened form of the SF-36: It has been used for many years as an instrument to evaluate quality of life in different diseases (Jenkinson and Layte 1997).

The questions were then adapted to the main known complaint problems from patients with lymphedema.

We added two more questions to evaluate the possible burden caused by the amount of time that was needed for conservative therapy and the impairment of wearing compression garments.

In order to guarantee an objective observation, we first tested the questionnaire for comprehensibility and suitability. Six patients (three males and three females), who were undergoing treatment and were not included in our study, were asked to fill out the questionnaires. The questionnaires were also tested by six members of the staff (two female nurses, a male nurse, one doctor, and a medical student). Every participant rated the questionnaire as comprehensible and had no problems answering the questions.

We separated the questionnaire into two major sections with the first part assessing the period prior to the surgery and the second part after lymphatic vessel transplantation. Each section addressed three major themes: physiological conditions, psychological conditions, and burden of conservative therapy.

Each question had five possible answers ranging from 1 (least harming with highest quality of life) to 5 (most harming with lowest quality of life). By utilizing a numerical scoring system, comparisons were accomplished by simply adding the number of points in the different parts of the survey for analysis. Scores were averaged for upper and lower limbs for each theme, standard error determined, and values used for before and after operation comparisons. All pre- and postoperative measurements and comparisons were evaluated with Mann-Whitney rank sum test, and significance was determined by $p \leq 0.001$ using SPSS.

4.5.1 Questions Regarding Physiological Conditions

This section includes four questions that assessed common problems for patients with lymphedema caused by the pressure of swollen tissue and skin: intensity of swelling, pain, paresthesias, and difficulty to work. The additional physiological question inquired about occurrence of skin infections and erysipelas.

4.5.2 Questions Regarding Psychological Conditions

This section contained four questions focusing on the social everyday and family life of the patients such as difficulties to get appropriate clothing, stigmatization, problems with the partner, and necessity to disclose the origin of the edema.

4.5.3 Questions Regarding Possible Burden of Conservative Therapy

This section consisted of two questions focusing on the burdens of conservative therapy including frequency of received manual lymph drainage and the impairment caused by wearing special compressive stockings.

References

Baumeister RGH, Seifert J, Hahn D (1981) Autotransplantation of Lymphatic Vessels. Lancet, Jan 17: 147

Jenkinson C, Layte R (1997) A shorter form health survey: can the SF-12 replicate results from the Sf-36 in longitudinal studies? J Public Health Med 19:179–209

Kleinhans E, Baumeister RG, Hahn D, Siuda S, Büll U, Moser E (1985) Evaluation of transport kinetics in lymphoscintigraphy: follow up study in patients with transplanted lymphatic vessels. Eur J Nucl Med 10:349–352

Koller M, Kussmann J (1995) Die Erfassung und Dokumentation der Lebensqualität nach Tumortherapie. Organspezifische Tumordokumentation. Springer, Berlin/Heidelberg

Kuhnke E (1976) Volumenbestimmung aus Umfangsmessungen. Folia Angiol 24:228–232

Kuhnke E (1978) Die Volumenbestimmung entrundeter Extremitäten aus Umfangsmessungen. Lymphologie 2:35–44

Lohrmann C, Foeldi E, Speck O, Langer M (2006) High-resolution MR lymphangiography in patients with primary and secondary lymphedema. AJR Am J Roentgenol 187:556–561

Lohrmann C, Foeldi E, Bartholoma JP, Langer M (2007) Magnetic resonance imaging of lymphatic vessels without image subtraction: a practicable imaging method for routine clinical practice? J Comput Assist Tomogr 31:303–308

Lohrmann C, Felmerer G, Foeldi E, Bartholoma JP, Langer M (2008) MR lymphangiography for the assessment of the lymphatic system in patients undergoing microsurgical reconstructions of lymphatic vessels. Microvasc Res 76:42–45

Michaely HJ, Kramer H, Attenberger U, Sourbron SP, Weckbach S, Reiser MF, Schoenberg SO (2007) Renal magnetic resonance angiography at 3.0 T: technical feasibility and clinical perspectives. Top Magn Reson Imaging 18:117–125

Notohamiprodjo M, Baumeister RGH, Jakobs TF, Bauner K, Boehm H, Horng A, Reiser MF, Glaser C, Herrmann KA (2009) MR-lymphangiography at 3.OT- a feasibility study. Eur Radiol 19:2771–2778

Notohamiprodjo M, Weiss M, Baumeister RGH, Sommer WH, Helck A, Crispin A, Reiser MF, Herrmann KA (2012) MR lymphangiography at 3.0.T: correlation with lymphoscintigraphy. Radiology 264:78–87

Partsch H, Stöberl C, Urbanek A, Wenzel-Hora BI (1988) Clinical use of indirect lymphography in different forms of leg edema. Lymphology 21:152–160

Springer S (2011) Veränderungen der Extremitätenvolumina und der Lebensqualität durch Lymphgefäßtransplantation bei Patienten mit Lymphödem. Inauguraldissertation LMU, München

Springer S, Koller R, Baumeister RGH, Frick A (2012) Changes in quality of life of patients with lymphedema after lymphatic vessel transplantation. Lymphology 44:65–71

Schoenberg SO, Rieger J, Weber CH, Michaely HJ, Waggershauser T, Ittrich C, Dietrich O, Reiser MF (2005) High-spatial-resolution MR angiography of renal arteries with integrated parallel acquisitions: comparison with digital subtraction angiography and US. Radiology 235:687–698

Weiss M, Baumeister RGH, Hahn K (2002) Post-therapeutic Lymphedema: scintigraphy before and after autologous lymph vessel transplantation 8 years of long-term follow-up Clin Nucl Med 27:788–792

Weiss M, Baumeister RGH, Hahn K (2003) Therapieplanung und Erfolgskontrolle der autologen Lymphgefäßtransplantation mittels nuklearmedizinischer Lymphabflussszintigraphie. Handchir Mikrochir Plast Chir 35:210–215

Weiss M, Baumeister RGH, Frick A, Wallmichrath J, Bartenstein P, Rominger A (2015a) Lymphedema of the upper limb evaluation of the functional outcome by dynamic imaging of lymph Kinetics after autologous lymph vessel transplantation. Clin Nucl Med 40:e117–e123

Weiss MF, Baumeister RGH, Zacherl MJ, Frick A, Bartenstein P, Rominger A (2015b) Microsurgical autologous lymph vessel transplantation: does harvesting lymphatic vessel grafts induce lymphatic transport disturbances in the donor limb? Handchir Mikrochir Plast Chir 47:359–364

Results of Reconstructive Lymph Vascular Surgery

5

5.1 Introductory Text

Between June 23, 1980, the first lymphatic vessel transplantation in man and January 2014 380 patients have been treated suffering from lymphedema due to a regional impairment of lymphatic flow. First results have been published in 1981 (Baumeister 1981; Baumeister et al. 1981a, b).

Most of the patients reported on previous interventions causing a local damage to the lymphatic transport system, mostly at the axilla or the groin or pelvic area.

215 patients showed a lymphedema of the upper limbs, and 155 patients suffered from lymphedema of the lower limbs. Ten patients had an edema of the penis and/or scrotum (Table 5.1).

5.2 Clinical Outcome in Treating Edemas of the Upper Limbs

Clinical outcome after lymphatic vessel transplantation was followed by volume measurement, lymphoscintigraphy, indirect lymphography, and quality of life assessment.

Several times, reports about actual results have been published using different evaluation methods. These are mentioned below according to the type of the follow-up method.

The actual report considers patients until January 2014.

Out of the 215 patients suffering from arm edemas, most of them, 207, were women with a history of mammary carcinoma. Only eight were man partly after mammary carcinoma too and some of them after Hodgkin treatment of Hodgkin disease. Only two patients suffered from a primary lymphedema (Table 5.2).

5.3 Volume Measurements

Volume measurements were performed using the method of Kuhnke (1976). First measurements were performed prior to surgery. These measurements represented the volume achieved by the treatment with conservative means. All patients had received complete decongestive treatment (CDT) during a minimum period of 6 months. Most of the patients had undergone this kind of treatment for years. In an earlier study, the mean duration of edema prior to surgery was about 7 years.

The first publication consisted of 36 patients, all except one with postmastectomy edemas.

The mean age of the postmastectomy edema patients was 56 years, ranging from 40 to 77 years. The mean interval between mastectomy and lymphatic grafting was 10 years, ranging from 17 months to 20 years. The mean interval between the onset of edema and lymphatic grafting was 8 years, ranging from 12 months to 20 years.

The mean arm volume of 3268 cm^3 preoperatively decreased to 2509 cm^3 2 weeks after grafting and came down to 2436 cm^3 about 2 years later. Sixteen patients with a follow-up of more than 3 years showed a mean decrease to 2195 cm^3. Three years after surgery, the volumes reached an order of magnitude almost similar to those of normal arms. Over the years, the decrease in volume was not only maintained but showed further decline. The reduction reached a level of 80 % in patients with a follow-up of at least 3 years. In all groups, the stated decrease was highly significant ($p < 0.001$) (Baumeister and Siuda 1990).

In 2003, the results in 127 arm edemas were published. There, the mean arm volume of 3368 cm^3 preoperatively decreased to 2567 cm^3 around 2 weeks after grafting and was 2625 cm^3 after a mean follow-up period of 2.6 years. The reduction in volume difference to the contralateral arm with a volume of 2224 cm^3 was about two third (Baumeister and Frick 2003).

Through January 2014 in 214 out of the 215 patients with arm edemas, volume measurements were performed. In one patient there was no contralateral arm present.

The mean arm volume of the normal contralateral side was 2262 ± 36 cm^3. The volume of the affected arm of 3288 ± 58 cm^3 preoperatively decreased to 2561 ± 39 cm^3

R.G.H. Baumeister, *Reconstructive Lymph Vascular Surgery*, DOI 10.1007/978-3-319-31647-5_5

Table 5.1 Patients treated by autogenous lymphatic vessel transplantation between June 1980 and January 2014

Autogenous lymphatic vessel transplantation	
6.1980–1.2014	
$n = 380$	
Upper limbs	215
Lower limbs	155
Penis and scrotum	10

Table 5.2 Gender and type of patients suffering from lymphedemas of the upper limbs treated by autogenous lymphatic vessel transplantation between June 1980 and January 2014

Autogenous lymphatic vessel transplantation	
6.1980–1.2014	
Edemas of the upper limbs	
$n = 215$	
Female	207
Male	8
Primary	2
Secondary	213

Table 5.3 Volume measurements in patients with arm lymphedema prior to lymphatic vessel transplantation, after hospital dismissal, and after a mean follow-up period of 2.5 years compared to the normal contralateral arm

Autogenous lymphatic vessel transplantation in edemas of the upper limbs					
Volumes: $\text{cm}^3\left(\bar{x}, s\bar{x}\right)$					
$n = 214$					
Normal	Preop	Postop Hosp. dism.	Postop 2.5 years	p (pre/post) Hosp. dism.	p (pre/post) 2.5 years
2262 ± 36	3288 ± 58	2561 ± 39	2634 ± 46	<0.001	<0.001

around 2 weeks after grafting and was 2634 ± 46 cm^3 after a mean follow-up period of 2.5 years. Both differences are highly significant ($p<0.001$) (Table 5.3, Fig. 5.1).

Of specific interest are the changes in volume in relation to the original volume difference between the normal and the affected arm.

Regarding the 214 patients, presenting two arms, reduction in the volume difference was seen in 204 patients after a mean follow-up period of 2.5 years after lymphatic vessel transplantation. Five percent showed a minimal reduction of up to 25 %. Forty-four patients showed a reduction between 25 and 50 %. A reduction of more than 50 % was seen in 149 patients, representing more than two third of the patients. Sixty-eight out of them had a reduction between 50 and 75 %, and more than 75 % reduction was seen in 81 patients (Tables 5.3 and 5.4; Fig. 5.2).

Long-term effect of treatment is the most important factor for the patient. We grouped the patients according to minimal follow-up periods. It was shown that the effect of diminishing the volume is constant over the years with a tendency to further improvement (Table 5.5, Fig. 5.3).

5.4 Nuclear Medical Investigations

All patients underwent lymphoscintigraphies prior to surgery. The examination included the leg provided for harvesting and the edematous extremity. If the patient agrees, we also check the postoperative status.

Figure 5.4 shows the follow-up of lymphoscintigraphies in a 55-year-old patient suffering from a secondary lymphedema of the left arm after mammary carcinoma before and 2, 4, and 6 years after lymphatic vessel transplantation. Prior to surgery, no activity is seen in the axilla and only a diffuse dispersion at the upper arm. After reconstruction, activity is seen corresponding to the course of the lymphatic grafts (see insert), demonstrating the transport of lymph within the grafts. The lymphatic transport index is

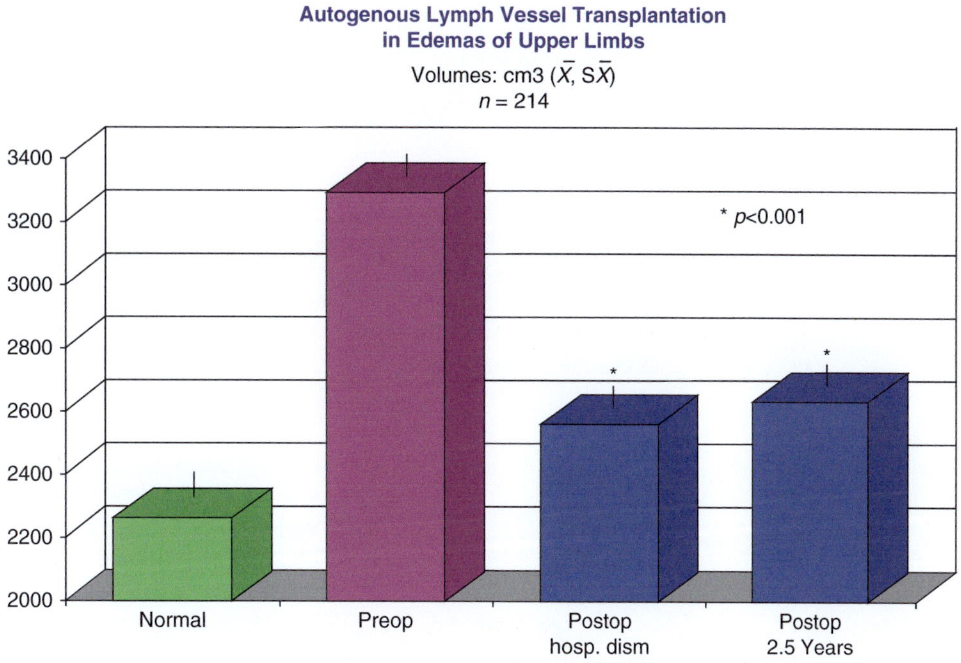

Fig. 5.1 Volume measurements in patients with arm lymphedema prior to lymphatic vessel transplantation, after hospital dismissal, and after a mean follow-up period of 2.5 years compared to the normal contralateral arm

Table 5.4 Changes in volume differences in arm lymphedema compared to the contralateral arm after lymphatic vessel transplantation

Changes in volume differences in edematous upper limbs after lymphatic vessel transplantation		
Difference: affected versus healthy extremity		
$n = 214$		
Mean follow-up period: 2.5 years		
	n	Percentage
Increase	10	5
Reduction		
<25 %	11	5
25–50 %	44	20
50–75 %	68	32
>75 %	81	38

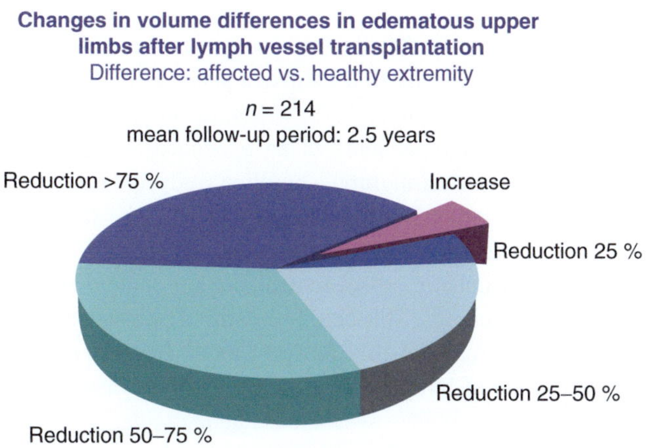

Fig. 5.2 Changes in volume differences in arm lymphedema compared to the contralateral arm after lymphatic vessel transplantation

diminished after the reconstruction, indicating the improvement in lymphatic transport.

At different time points, the transport of lymph was followed by investigators of the Department of Nuclear Medicine at the Ludwig Maximilians University Munich.

The first investigation dated from 1985. The survey included the upper and lower extremities as well.

In 23 patients with lymphatic vessel grafts, the first medical control was undertaken at the end of hospitalization, i.e., 7–14 days after transplantation at that time. The average decrease of TI was 5.9 points. It was reduced from 31.1 points before to 25.2 points after transplantation. The corresponding volumes decreased from 3435 to 2547 ml. The changes in TI and volume were significant ($p < 0.05$). By comparison, the mean volume in the healthy contralateral side was 1854 ml (Kleinhans et al. 1985).

Table 5.5 Long-term follow-up after lymphatic vessel transplantation in arm edemas

Autogenous lymphatic vessel transplantation in edemas of the upper limbs

Volumes: cm^3 $(\bar{x}, s\bar{x})$

Minimal follow-up periods

	n	Normal	Preop	Postop	Preop	p pre/post	p pre/post
				Hosp. dism.	Last meas.	Hosp. dism.	Last meas.
>1 year	118	2190 ± 46	3230 ± 76	2531 ± 51	2638 ± 64	<0.001	<0.001
>3 years	55	2035 ± 72	3044 ± 104	2399 ± 73	2461 ± 193	<0.001	<0.001
>6 years	23	2000 ± 78	3116 ± 165	2405 ± 117	2344 ± 130	<0.001	<0.001
>8 years	17	1899 ± 79	2855 ± 126	2273 ± 122	2220 ± 125	<0.001	<0.001

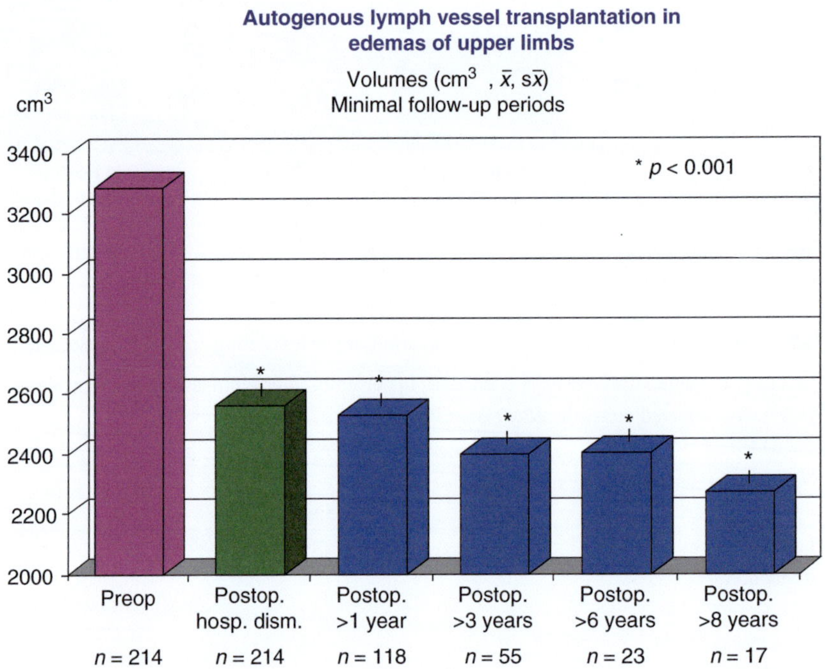

Fig. 5.3 Long-term follow-up after lymphatic vessel transplantation in arm edemas

A series of patients with edemas of the upper and lower extremities and patients with primary and secondary lymphedemas was investigated in a study consisting of 20 patients (17 females and 3 males). A preoperative baseline study was compared to postoperative follow-up investigations for a period of 7 years. The reason for microsurgical lymphatic vessel transplantation was in four patients a primary and in 16 patients a secondary lymphedema. In 12 cases, the transplantation side was at the upper extremity and in eight cases at the lower limb.

In 17 out of 20 patients, the lymphatic function improved after autologous lymphatic vessel transplantation compared to preoperative findings, as verified by visual improvement of lymph drainage and decrease of numeric transport index. In five cases the vessel graft could be directly visualized. In these patients with scintigraphic visualization of the vessel grafts, the transport index decreased to a significantly greater extent compared to the preoperative baseline study. Only three patients did not benefit from microsurgical treatment (Weiss et al. 1996).

Specifically patients with arm edemas were investigated in a study with a long-term follow-up of 8 years. Twelve patients were included (age range, 32–73 years; mean age, 56 years) with secondary lymphedema of an upper extremity. All of them underwent a scintigraphic baseline study and follow-up study for a period of 8 years after microsurgical treatment.

In 11 of 12 patients, lymphatic function improved after autologous lymphatic vessel transplantation compared with preoperative findings. This could be verified by a statistically significant decrease of the transport index (p<0.01), clear demonstration of lymph nodes, and less diffuse distribution pattern of the Tc-99 m-labeled nanocolloids. In three patients, the vessel grafts could be detected by scintigraphy (Weiss et al. 2002).

The most recent study about patients suffering from arm lymphedema consisted of 177 patients (172 females, five

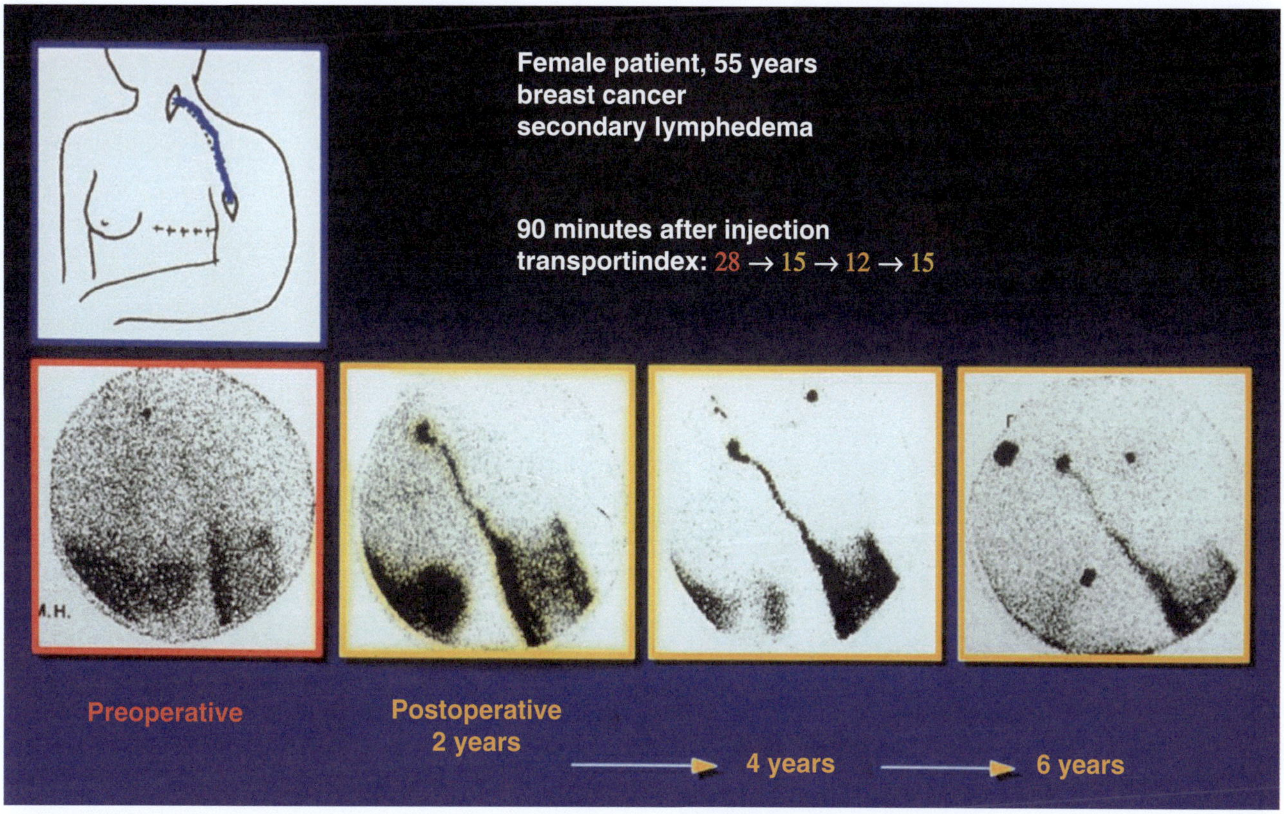

Fig. 5.4 Example of improvement of lymphatic transport, demonstrated by lymphoscintigraphy and calculated by lymphatic transport index in a 55-year-old patient suffering from a secondary lymphedema of the left arm with a follow-up of 6 years

males; median age, 56 years, range 12–84 years) after lymphatic vessel transplantation in the upper extremity. For correlation of scintigraphic data versus reduction of volume (RV) surplus, measurements at four different time points were performed as follows: preoperatively (T0), within 2 weeks after Tx (T1), 6–12 months after Tx (T2), and 32–38 months after Tx (T3). An additional long-term follow-up after at least 8 years was available in some cases.

The maximum individual postoperative observation period was 19 years. In 169 of 177 cases, lymphedema had been caused by treatment of breast cancer (mastectomy, $n=103/169$; breast preserving, $n=66/169$; and/or radiation therapy, $n=130/177$), but two patients presented with primary lymphedema. The remaining six cases of lymphatic disorders were caused by treatment of malignant melanoma, Hodgkin lymphoma, axillary Ewing sarcoma, non-Hodgkin lymphoma, hemangioma, or abscess removal.

At T1, the mean RV of the affected limb was 73 %, and the mean improvement of transport index (TI) was 28 %. At T2, the RV was 64 % and the TI was 23 %. And at T3, the RV was 63 % and the TI was 25 %.

Long-term follow-up after at least 8 years (T4, range, 9–19.2; mean, 14.1 years) was available in 19 of 177 patients in whom persistent improvement in the scintigraphic data (25 % decrease in TL) was confirmed by a mean clinical RV of 68 %. The mean overall correlation was by a factor of 2.64 (Weiss et al. 2015) (Fig. 5.5).

5.5 Radiological Investigations

To prove the patency of the lymphatic grafts by direct visualization is difficult. Investigations with oily contrast medium like Lipiodol® need to sacrifice at least on lymphatic channel. Furthermore it does harm to the lymphatic vessels and lymph nodes.

Using water-soluble contrast medium is less dangerous; however mostly only lymphatic vessels close to the side of administration of the contrast agent are visualized. Therefore, only in single patients, it was possible to prove the patency of lymphatic grafts in the upper extremity more than 10 years after surgery (Baumeister et al. 2011).

Figure 5.6 gives an example of a 41-year-old patient at a long term follow up after reconstructive surgery. After mastectomy, axillary dissection, and radiation therapy, she had developed lymphedema of the left arm which was treated by autogenous lymphatic grafts 4 years later. Twelve years after lymphatic grafting, the indirect lymphography showed the patent graft.

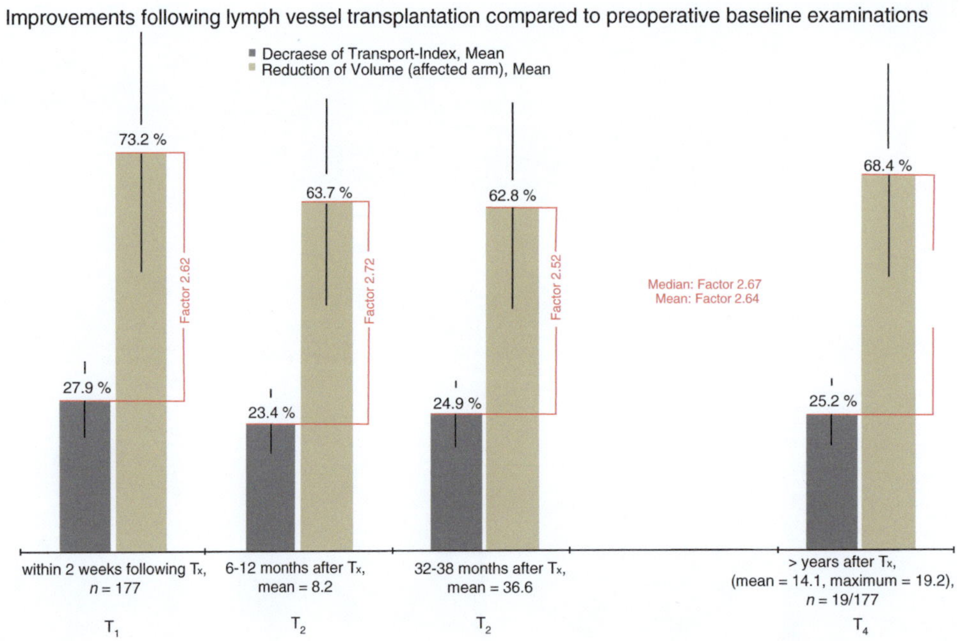

Fig. 5.5 Comparison of improvement regarding lymphatic transport index and reduction of volume after lymphatic reconstruction in arm edemas in contrast to baseline investigation, 2 weeks, 6–12 months, 32–38 months, and more than 8 years after surgery (From: Nuclear med 2015! © Wolters Kluwer Health)

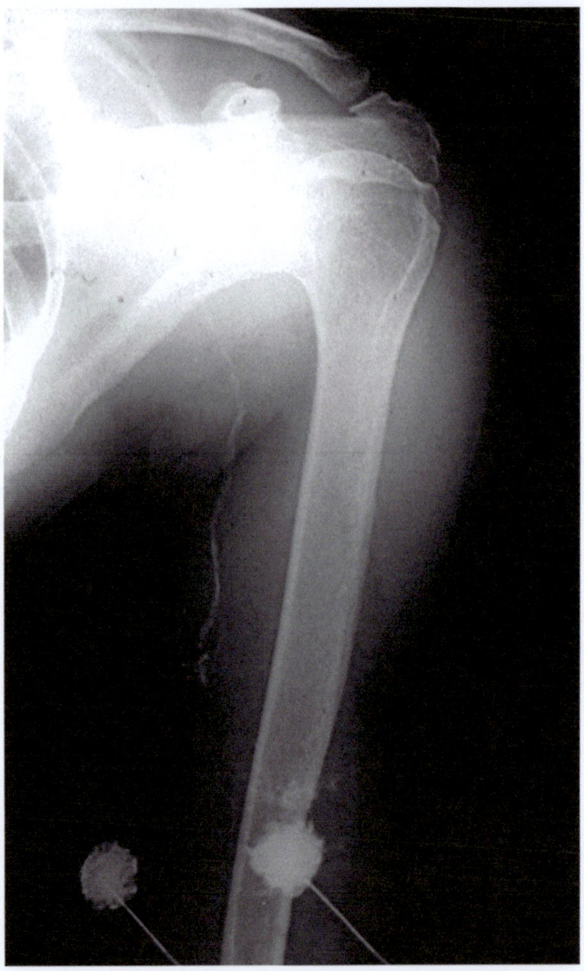

Fig. 5.6 Indirect lymphography using water-soluble contrast medium (Isovist®) 12 years after lymphatic grafting showing the graft on the medial aspect of the upper arm, bypassing the left axilla

Since lymphoscintigraphy shows a good correlation to radiological findings, the patency may be also estimated indirectly also by lymphoscintigraphy. When activity is seen clearly along the route of the graft, this might be a sufficient proof for a patent graft (Weiss et al. 2015).

5.6 Quality of Life Studies

Quality of life studies were performed consisting of 212 patients who were treated between 1983 and 2007 (Springer 2011, Springer et al. 2012).

Experiencing a response rate of 73 % of the questioned patients, 70 patients with arm edemas could be assessed. The questions touched the physiological and psychological conditions and the burden of the conservative treatment.

The average score for physiological condition prior to surgery was 13.8 ± 0.4 (mean ± SEM) points.

After surgery, the average score fell to 9.1 ± 0.3. This was a significant positive change in quality of life of 4.7 ($p \leq 0.001$) (Fig. 5.7).

For patients with arm lymphedema, the average score for psychological condition prior to surgery was 15.6 ± 0.5 (mean ± SEM) points.

After surgery, the average score fell to 11 ± 0.5. This was a significant positive change in quality of life of 4.6 points ($p \leq 0.001$) (Fig. 5.8).

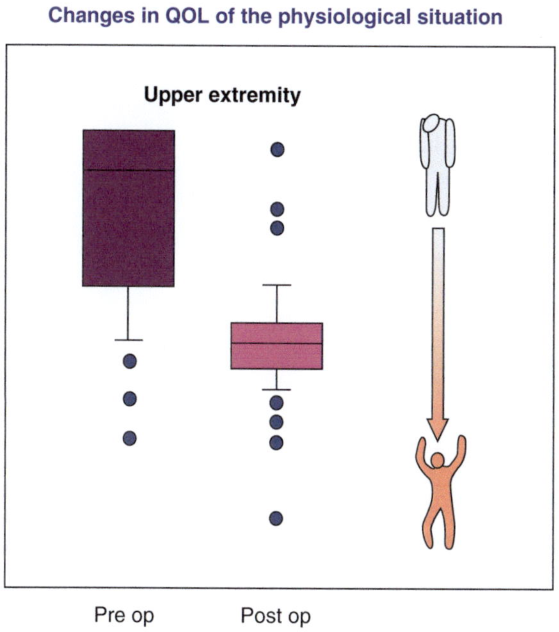

Fig. 5.7 Quality of life regarding physiological conditions, values for patients with lymphedema of the arm before and after lymphatic vessel transplantation. Data presented as the 25th to 75th percentiles (*boxes*) with mean (*line in box*), SE (*bars*), and outlying points (*circles*). QOL improves with decrease of points

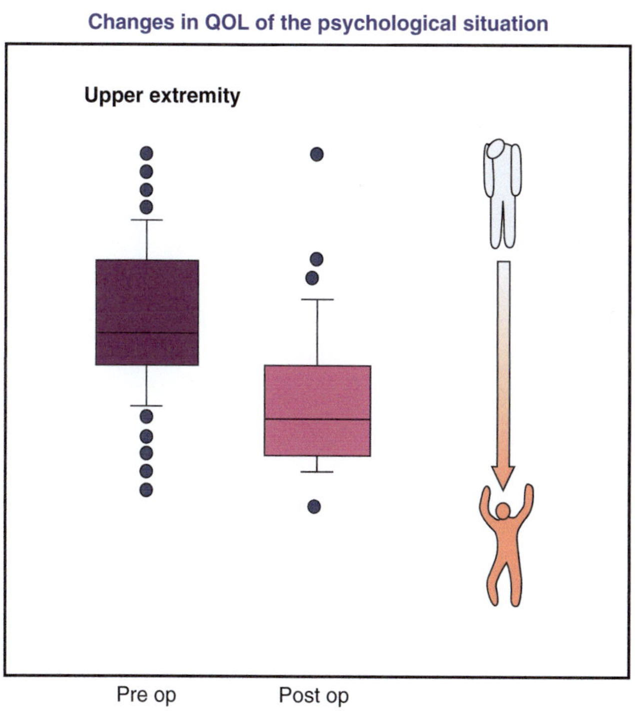

Fig. 5.8 Quality of life regarding psychological conditions, values for patients with lymphedema of the arm before and after lymphatic vessel transplantation. Data presented as the 25th to 75th percentiles (*boxes*) with mean (*line in box*), SE (*bars*), and outlying points (*circles*). QOL improves with decrease of points

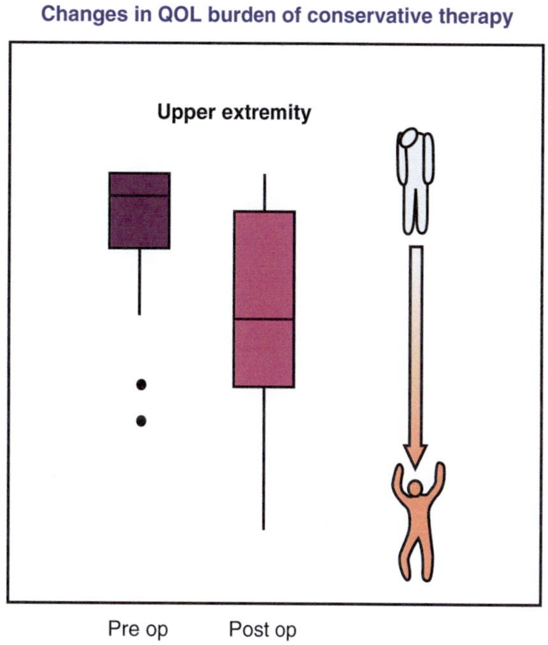

Fig. 5.9 Quality of life regarding the burden of conservative therapy, values for patients with lymphedema of the arm before and after lymphatic vessel transplantation. Data presented as the 25th to 75th percentile (*boxes*) with mean (*line in box*), SE (*bars*), and outlying points (*circles*). QOL improves with decrease of points

For patients with arm lymphedema, the average score for burden of conservative treatment prior to surgery was 9 ± 0.2 (mean ± SEM) points.

After surgery, the average score fell to 6.4 ± 0.3 points. This is a significant positive change in quality of life of 2.6 points ($p \leq 0.001$) (Fig. 5.9).

5.7 Examples

The examples show different types of lymphedemas and different time intervals between reconstructive surgery and the time of documentation. For patients with arm edema, the condition of the hand is of utmost importance as well as the question if compression garments have to be worn. Important for the patients is also the feeling of an elevated pressure within the tissue. Regression or disappearance of the feeling of compression is the first observation by the patient after reconstruction of lymphatic flow. Reducing the volume toward a normal size with lymphatic reconstruction alone is possible at best in moderate edemas with predominance of fluid content (Figs. 5.10, 5.11, and 5.13). In advanced lymphedema with high amount of additional fat deposits, either the patient is content with the reduction in size and molestation (Fig. 5.12) or additional reduction of fat is performed in a secondary procedure, once lymphatic outflow is corrected successfully.

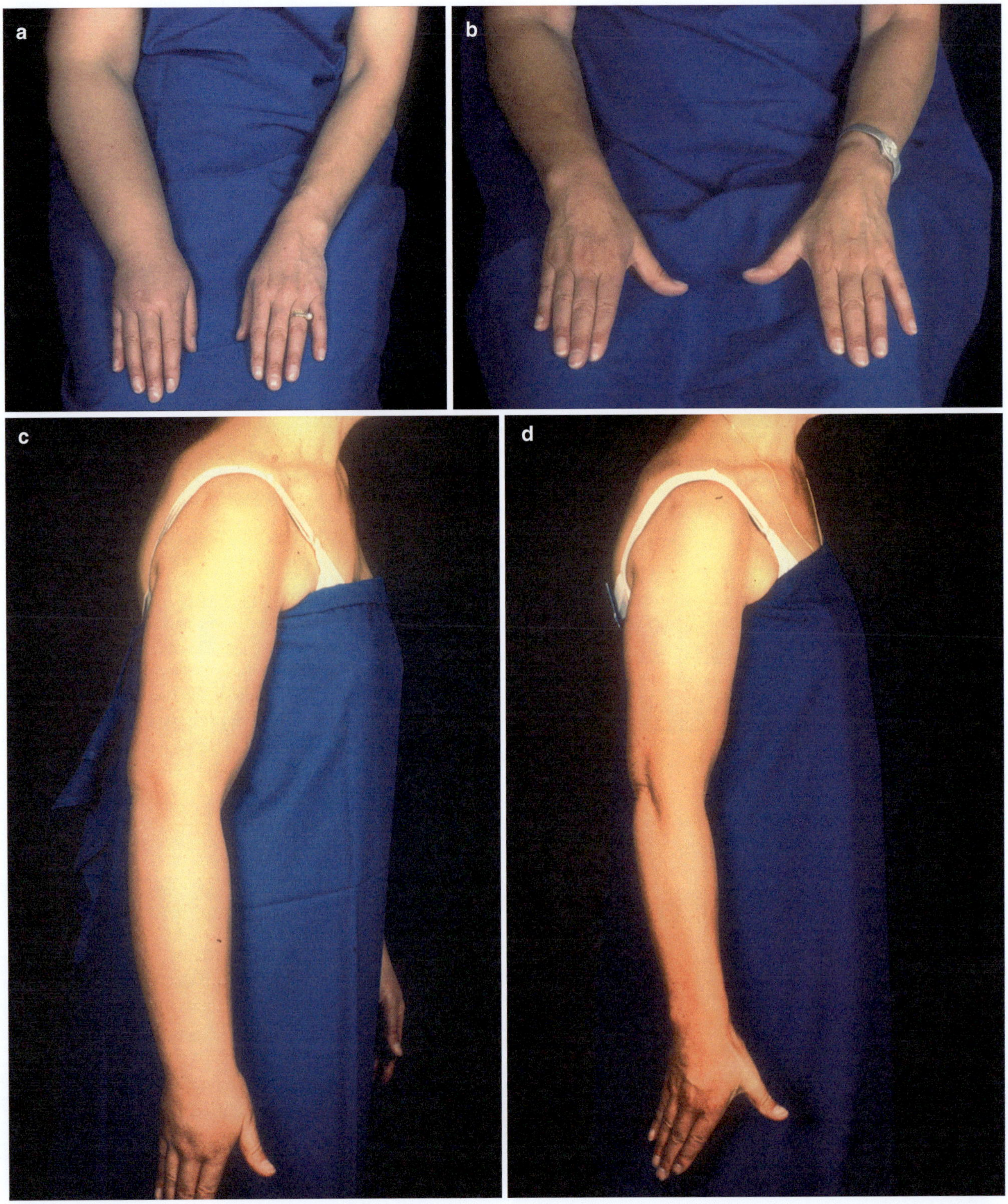

Fig. 5.10 (**a**) A 50-year-old patient, 6 years after axillary dissection in the course of mammary carcinoma treatment on the right axilla. (**b**) 9 months after lymphatic vessel transplantation, of specific importance for the patients is to get the hand free of edema without additional treatment. (**c**) Lateral view, prior to surgery. (**d**) After lymphatic reconstruction

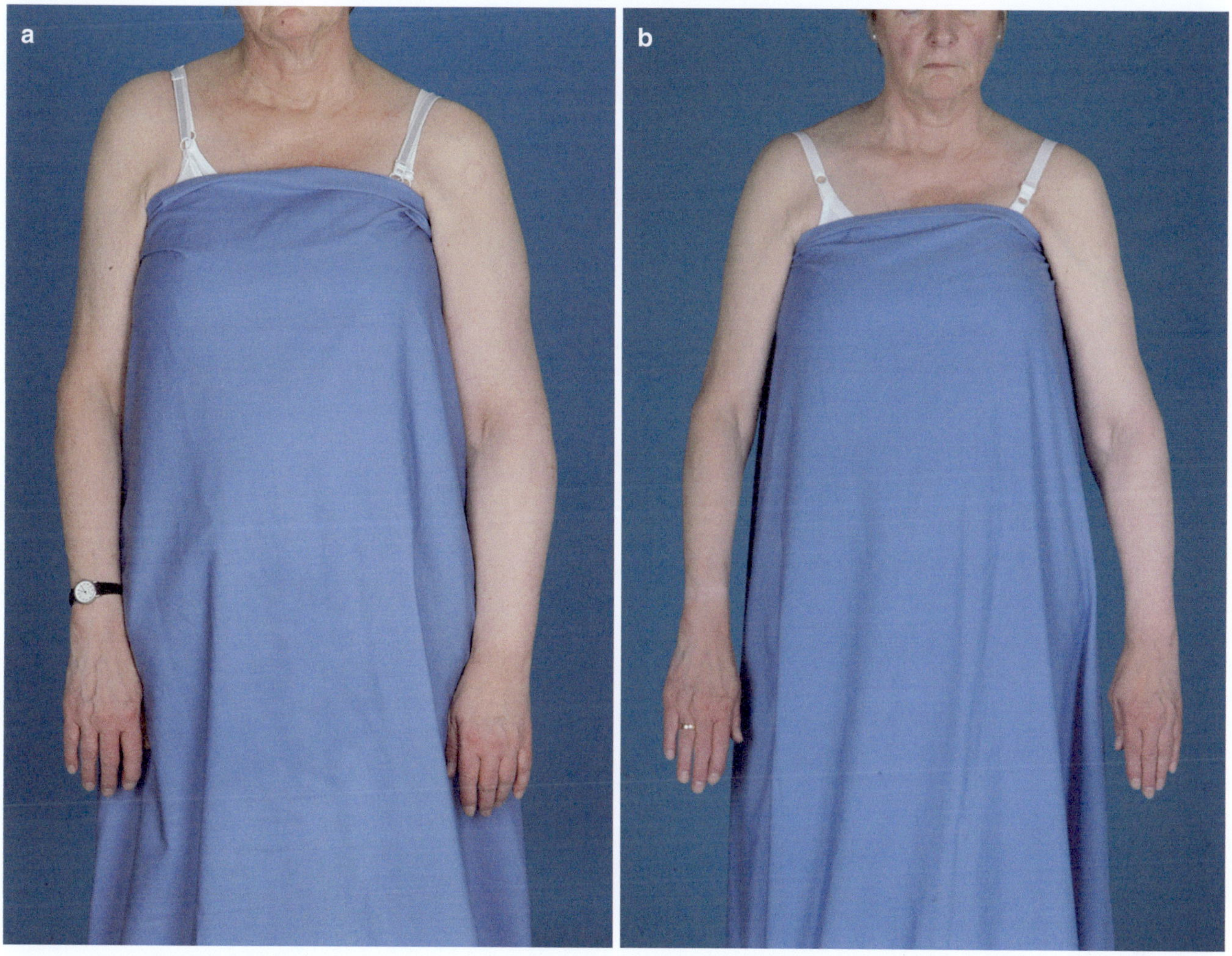

Fig. 5.11 (**a**) A 64-year-old patient, 7 years after breast conservative treatment, radiation, and chemotherapy and 6 years of edema and conservative treatment. (**b**) 2 years after reconstructive surgery, bypassing the left axilla (© Baumeister)

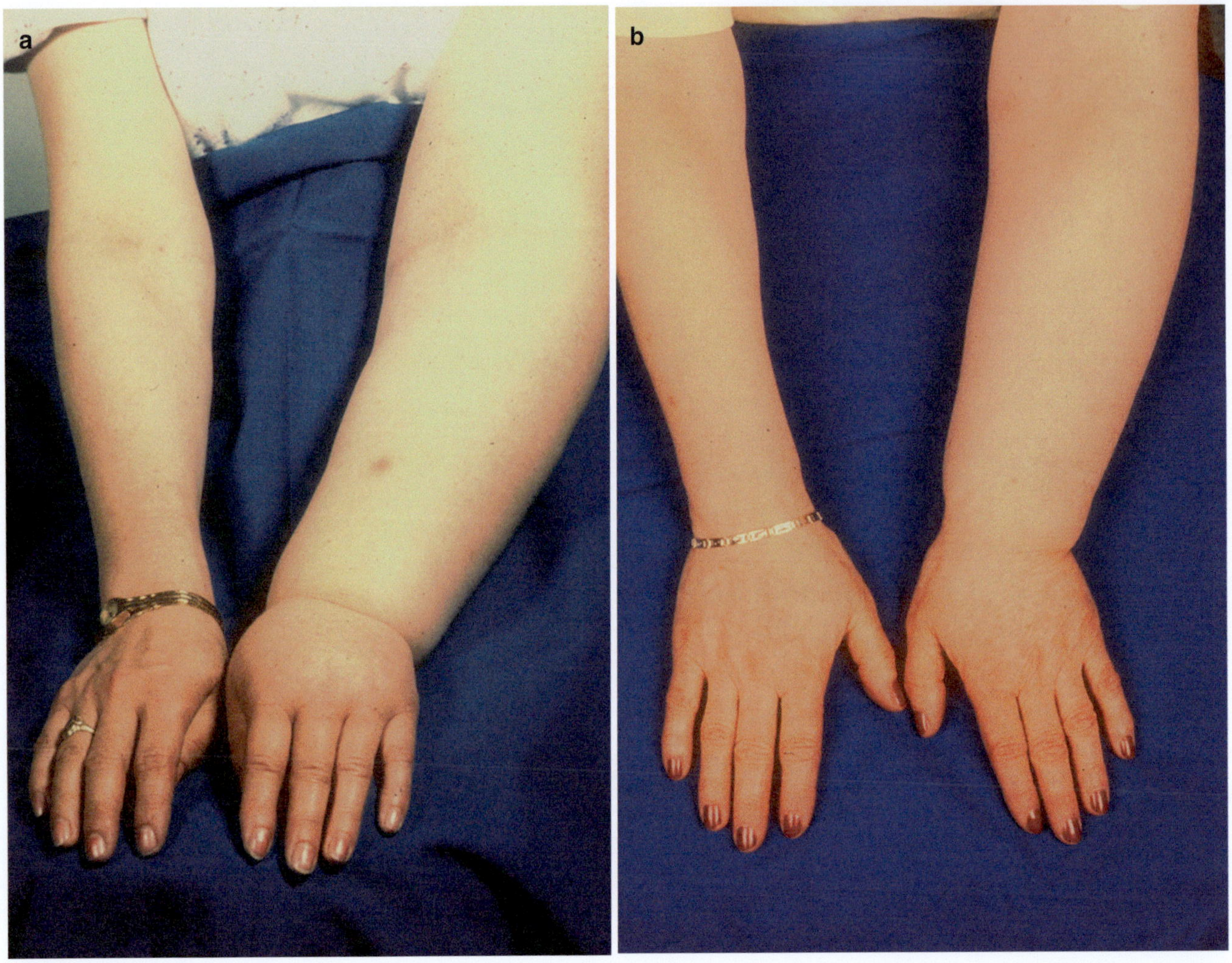

Fig. 5.12 (**a**) A 41-year-old patient, advanced secondary arm lymphedema 4 years after mastectomy, axilla dissection, and radiation therapy. (**b**) 10 years after lymphatic vessel transplantation, no further therapy, today secondary liposuction would be recommended for the forearm (© Baumeister)

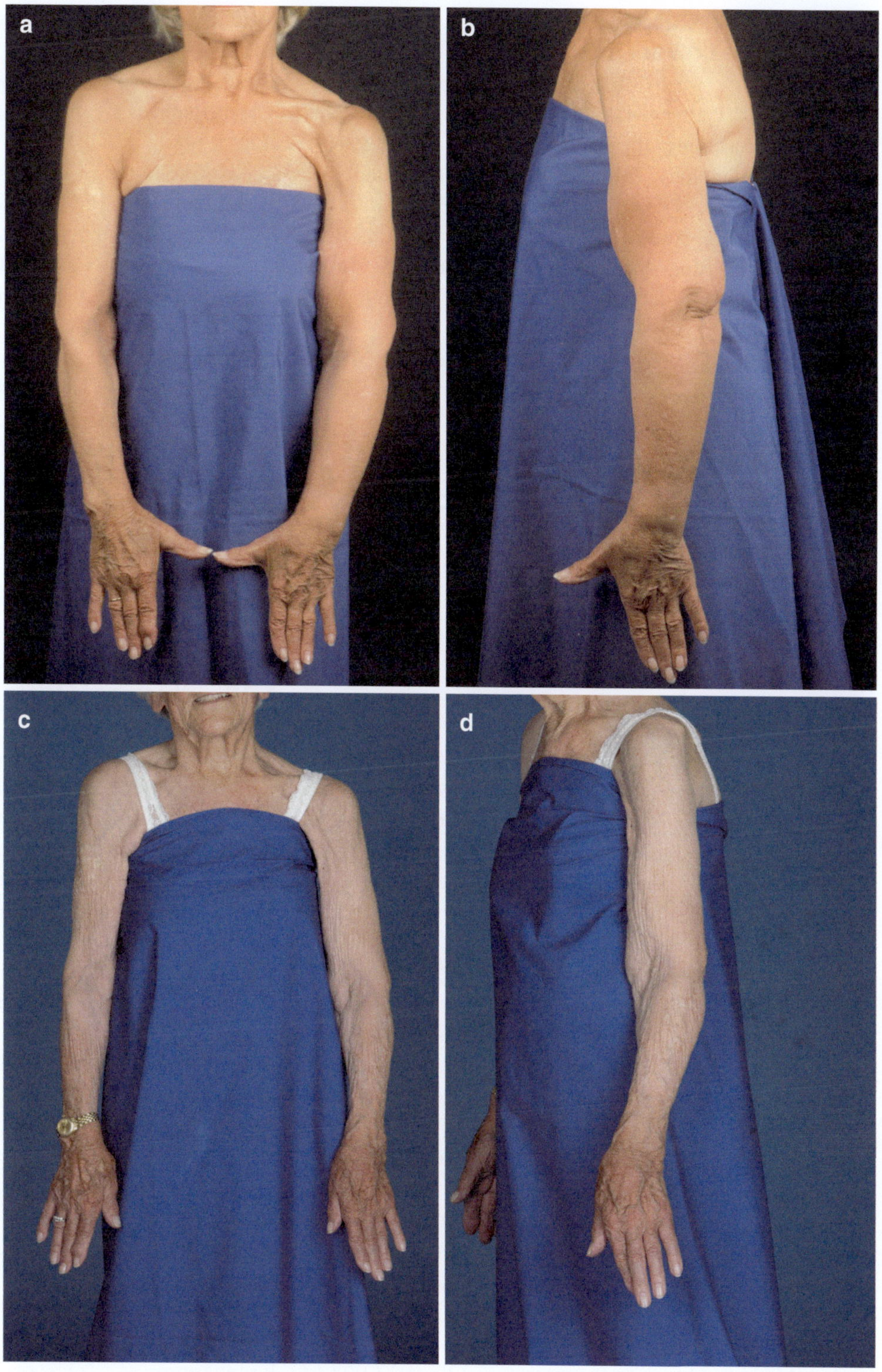

Fig. 5.13 (**a**) A 75-year-old patient, 23 years after mastectomy and axillary dissection, secondary lymphedema left arm conservative treatment (front view). (**b**) Lateral view. (**c**) 14 years after lymphatic vessels transplantation bypassing the axilla without any additional therapy (front view). (**d**) (lateral view)

5.8 Clinical Outcome in Treating Edemas of the Lower Limbs

Clinical outcome after lymphatic vessel transplantation was followed by volume measurement, lymphoscintigraphy, indirect lymphography, MR lymphography, and quality of life assessment.

At several time points, reports about actual results have been published using different evaluation methods. These are mentioned below according to the type of the follow-up method.

The actual report considers patients until January 2014.

Autogeneous lymph vessel transplantation	
6.1980–1.2014	
Edemas of lower limbs	
$n = 155$	
Female	117
Male	38
Primary	50
Secondary	105

5.9 Volume Measurement

The first publication considered 18 patients with lymphedema of the lower extremity. Four edemas were of primary, 13 of iatrogenic, and one of traumatic origin. Twelve of the patients were adults and six were children or adolescents. The mean age of the adults was 38 years, ranging from 23 to 63 years.

The statistical evaluation of treatment in the lower extremities only included the adult patients. The volumes of the unaffected contralateral legs in adults remain constant, making them more comparable as opposed to measurements undertaken in children, in whom normal leg volumes vary considerably during growth.

In 12 adult patients, a significant reduction in volume after 14 days was seen. The preoperative volume with 11,413 cm^3 came down to 8920 cm^3 and after 1 year to 9432 cm^3 in eight patients. The decrease was significant to values of $p=0.01$ and 0.05, respectively (Baumeister 1990; Baumeister and Siuda 1990).

In 2003 the results in 81 adult patients with leg edema were published. The volume was reduced from 13,098 to 10,578 cm^3 ($p \leq 0.001$) and to 10,692 cm^3 after 4 years ($p \leq 0.001$). The original mean volume of the healthy contralateral leg was 9371 cm^3 (Baumeister and Frick 2003).

Through January 2014, 145 adult patients with unilateral leg edema have been treated.

The mean volume of the normal contralateral side was 9447 ± 157 cm^3. The mean volume of the affected lower extremity of 12,784 ± 258 cm^3 preoperatively decreased to 10,404 ± 205 cm^3 around 2 weeks after grafting and was 10,987 ± 230 cm^3 after a mean follow-up period of 1.9 years. The differences are highly significant ($p<0.001$) (Table 5.6) (Fig. 5.14).

Looking to the relative variation in volume in relation to all adults patients, in 15 patients the natural progression of lymphedema could not be retarded. Also in another 10 %, the decline in volume was less than 25 %. However in 64 % of the patients, the reduction in volume difference was more than 50 % (Table 5.7 and Fig. 5.15).

In the long-term follow-up, we saw significant reduction also in the group of patients with a minimal follow-up period of 4 years.

After more than 8 years follow-up, there was no significant reduction to state. Only a lasting tendency of reduction was seen (Table 5.6, Fig. 5.16).

The results show that in the lower extremities, it is more difficult to achieve constant results compared to the upper extremities.

5.10 Nuclear Medical Investigations

The transport of lymph has been followed by investigators of the Department of Nuclear Medicine at the Ludwig Maximilians University Munich at several points of time.

The first investigation dated from 1985. The survey included the upper and lower extremities as well.

In 23 patients with lymphatic vessel grafts, the first medical control was done at 7–14 days after transplantation. The average decrease of transport index (TI) was 5.9 points. It decreased from 31.1 points before to 25.2 points after transplantation. The corresponding volumes decreased from 3435 to 2547 ml. Changes in TI and volume were significant ($p<0.05$). The mean volume, on the other hand, in the healthy contralateral side was 1854 ml (Kleinhans et al. 1985).

A further publication in 1996 reported about eight patients with lymphedemas of the lower extremities. Four of them had a primary or a secondary lymphedema. Seven out of eight patients showed a significant decrease of the lymphatic transport index which means a significant improvement of lymphatic transport after microsurgical lymphatic vessels transposition. In two of the patients, the transposed lymphatic vessels were visualized directly (Weiss et al. 1996).

As an example, the follow-up of lymphoscintigraphy in 36-year-old patient suffering from a primary lymphedema of the left leg before and 2, 4, and 6 years after lymphatic vessel transposing is displayed. The grafts have been harvested on the right thigh (see graphic insert above). In the preoperative lymphoscintigraphy, transport of lymph is

Table 5.6 Volumes of the lower extremities in unilateral lymphedemas before and after lymphatic reconstructive surgery compared to the normal contralateral leg in adults

Autogenous lymphatic vessel transplantation in unilateral edemas of the lower limbs in adults

Volumes: cm^3($\bar{x}$, $s\bar{x}$)

$n = 145$

Normal	Preop	Postop Hosp. dism.	Postop 1.9 years	p (pre/post) Hosp. dism.	p (pre/post) 1.9. years
9447 (±157)	12,784 (±258)	10,404 (±205)	10,987 (±230)	<0.001	<0.001

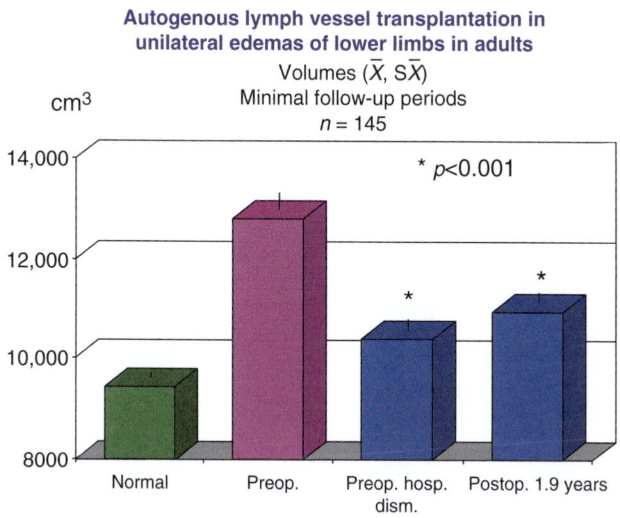

Fig. 5.14 Mean volumes of the lower extremities in adult patients, comparing contralateral leg with pre- and postoperative status of edematous limb

clearly demonstrated at the harvesting side. On the left side, no activity at all is seen despite injection of the radiopharmaceutical on both sides. After reconstructive surgery, injection of the radiopharmaceutical was performed only on the left side. Lymphatic flow (partly disseminated) is now seen up to the groin on the left side. Below the activity in the bladder, above the symphysis, activity is crossing toward the right inguinal lymph nodes. Disseminated distribution of the activity on the affected left leg is diminished with the years. Activity along the route of the grafts is furthermore clearly seen together with the activity within the lymph nodes on the right side where no activity was administered. The lymphatic transport index is reduced indicating the improvement in lymphatic transport (Fig. 5.17).

5.11 Radiological Investigations

To prove the patency of the lymphatic grafts by direct visualization is difficult. Investigations with oily contrast medium like Lipiodol® need to sacrifice at least on lymphatic channel. Furthermore it does harm to the lymphatic vessels and lymph nodes.

Using water-soluble contrast medium is less dangerous; however mostly only lymphatic vessels close to the side of administration of the contrast agent are visualized. In single patients, however, it was possible to prove the patency of lymphatic grafts in the upper extremity more than 10 years after surgery (Baumeister et al. 2011).

Figure 5.18 shows the proof of patent lymphatic graft 10 years after transposing the lymphatic vessels from the left groin to the right thigh because of lymphedema of the left leg. Water-soluble contrast medium was injected on the distal part of the right thigh. The flow is demonstrated from the right affected side to the inguinal nodes on the left healthy side.

With the help of MRI lymphography, the small lymphatic vessels are displayed best near the central axis of the body within the machine. Proof of patency of lymphatic grafts which transverse the symphysis is therefore possible.

Also if radiological remonstration of patency is not possible on each patient because of technical and financial reasons, the example demonstrates the long-term patency of lymphatic autografts.

Figure 5.19 demonstrates a patent lymphatic graft which was transposed from the left leg to the right, edematous extremity 7 years before.

5.12 Quality of Life Studies

Quality of life studies were performed consisting of 212 patients who were treated between 1983 and 2007 (Springer 2011, Springer et al. 2012).

Experiencing a response rate of 63 % of the questioned patients, 68 patients with leg edemas could be assessed.

The questions touched the physiological and psychological conditions and the burden of the conservative treatment.

The average score for physiological condition prior to surgery was 12.3 ± 0.4 (mean ± SEM) points. After surgery, the average score fell to 9.1 ± 0.3. This was a significant positive change in quality of life of 4.7 ($p \leq 0.001$) (Fig. 5.20).

Table 5.7 Changes in volume difference in the unilateral leg lymphedemas after lymphatic vessel transplantation

Changes in volume differences in edematous lower limbs of adults after lymphatic vessel transplantation		
Difference: affected versus healthy extremity		
$n = 145$		
Mean follow-up period: 1.9 years		
	n	Percentage
Increase	15	10
Reduction		
<25 %	14	10
25–50 %	23	16
50–75 %	44	30
>75 %	49	34

Table 5.8 Volumes in unilateral edemas of the lower limbs after minimal follow-up periods of 1, 4, and 8 years following lymphatic reconstruction

Autogenous lymphatic vessel transplantation in unilateral edemas of the lower limbs in adults							
Volumes: cm^3 ($\bar{x}$, $s\bar{x}$)							
Minimal follow-up periods							
	n	Normal	Preop	Postop	Preop	p pre/post	p pre/post
				Hosp. dism.	Last meas.	Hosp. dism.	Last meas.
>1 year	57	9303 ± 225	12,977 ± 412	10,613 ± 332	11,422 ± 400	<0.001	<0.001
>4 years	19	8868 ± 367	12,153 ± 522	10,168 ± 386	11,153 ± 710	<0.001	<0.05
>8 years	11	8818 ± 507	12,041 ± 742	10,227 ± 544	11,385 ± 1002	<0.001	ns.

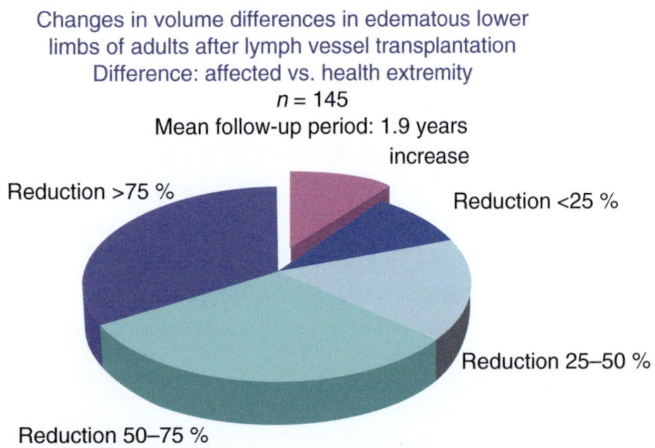

Fig. 5.15 Change in volume differences between affected and healthy lower extremities after lymphatic vessel transplantation

For patients with leg lymphedema, the average score for psychological condition prior to surgery was 13.6±0.5 (mean±SEM) points.

After surgery, the average score fell to 1.41±0.6. This was a significant positive change in quality of life of 1.6 points ($p \leq 0.001$) (Fig. 5.21).

For patients with leg lymphedema, the average score for burden of conservative treatment prior to surgery was 8.1±0.3 (mean±SEM) points.

After surgery, the average score fell to 7.9±0.3 points. This is a significant positive change in quality of life of 2.6 points ($p \leq 0.001$) (Fig. 5.22).

5.13 Examples

The example of a lymphedema of the whole lower extremity caused by a lymphatic obstacle within the pelvic area depicts a 70-year-old lady. Because of a corpus carcinoma, she underwent a radical operation together with a radiation therapy. Additionally lymph nodes at the right groin were removed. Two years later, she developed a lymphedema of the right leg which was treated by CDT for 12 years. Thereafter she underwent the microsurgical reconstruction. Three lymphatic collectors together with one side branch were transposed from the opposite leg and anastomosed with four ascending lymphatic collectors beneath the groin at the edematous limb. Figure 5.23a, b shows the preoperative situation. Figure 5.23c, d displays the situation 11 years after surgery.

The example of a lymphatic obstacle in the periphery of an extremity depicts the sequel of a surgical intervention at the knee in a 45-year-old man. The patient was operated on a Baker cyst on the right knee, followed by a subsequent infection.

Fig. 5.16 Volumes of the lower limbs in adults prior to lymphatic grafting and at minimal follow-up periods of 1, 4, and 8 years

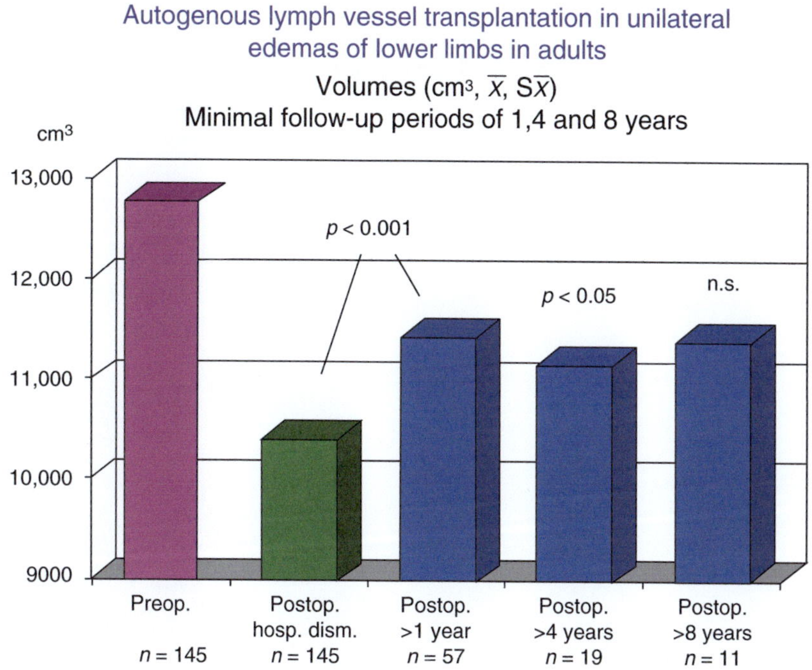

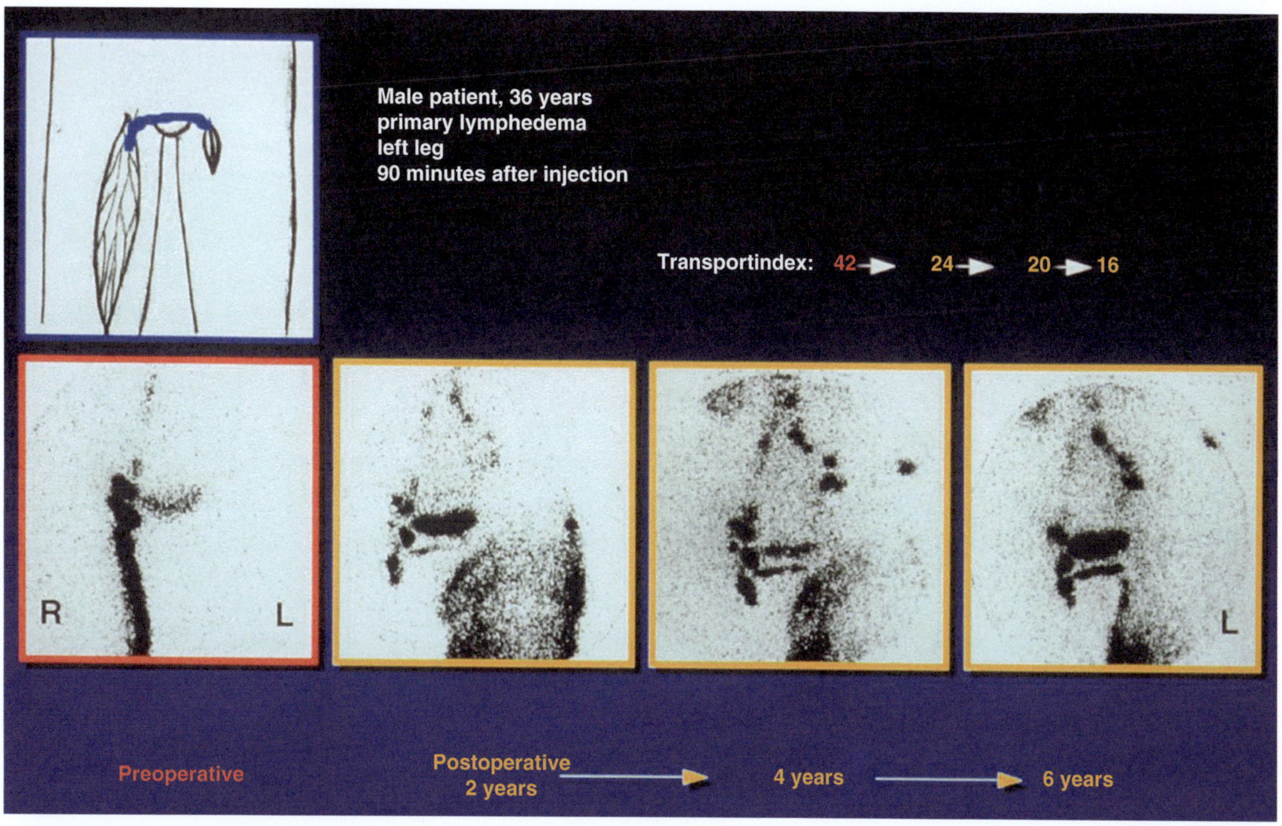

Fig. 5.17 Example of improvement in lymphatic transport, demonstrated by lymphoscintigraphy and calculated by lymphatic transport index in a 36-year-old patient suffering from a primary lymphedema of the left leg

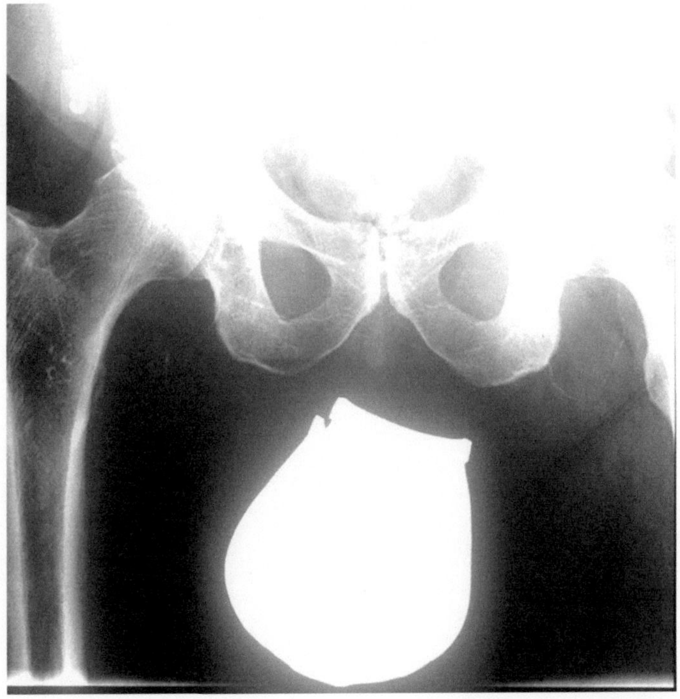

Fig. 5.18 Indirect lymphography using water-soluble contrast medium (Isovist®) 10 years after lymphatic grafting showing the graft running from right side of the patient toward the left side

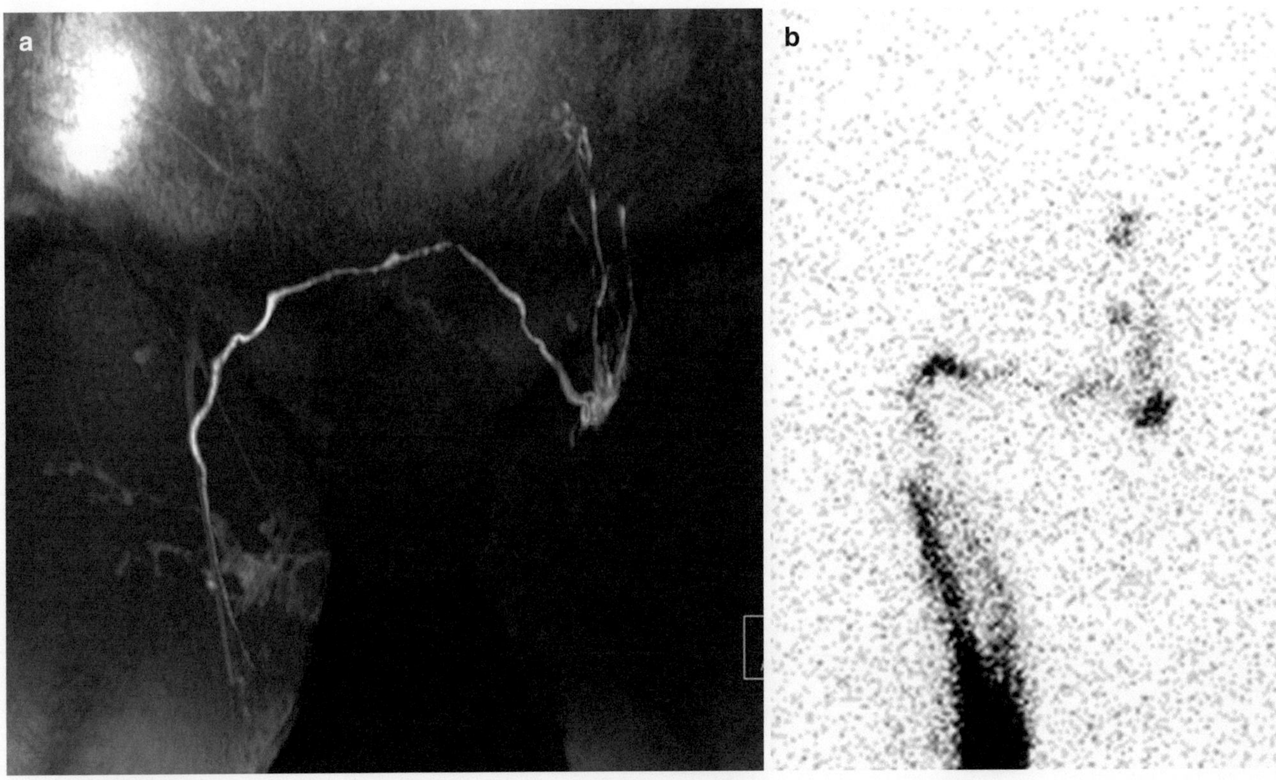

Fig. 5.19 (**a**) Patent lymphatic graft, transposed from the left side, anastomosed to ascending lymphatic collectors at the right side, 7 years follow-up. (**b**) Function and patency proved by lymphoscintigraphy at the same patient (injection only at the *right side*) (© Baumeister)

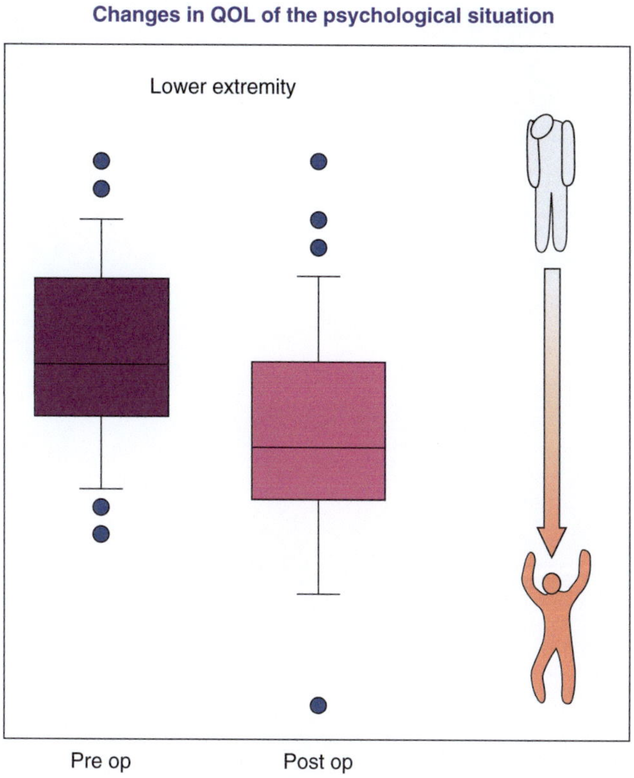

Fig. 5.20 Quality of life regarding the psychological situation (average scores, mean ± SEM, the lower the score, the better the quality of life) before and after lymphatic vessel transplantation in lymphedema of the lower extremity

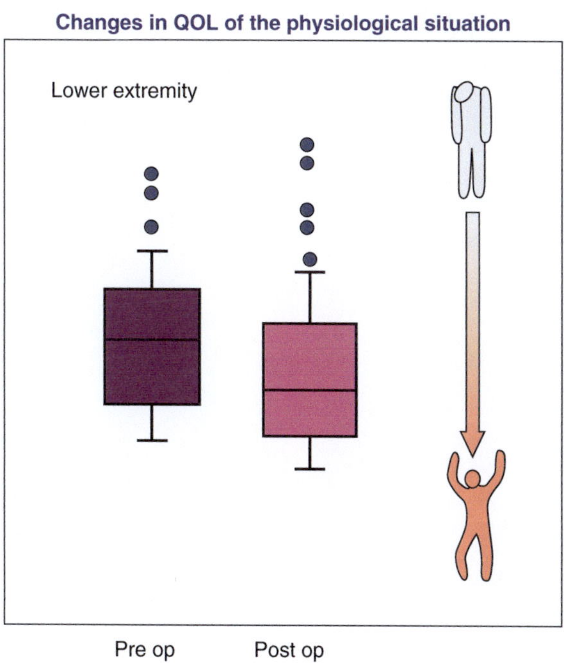

Fig. 5.21 Quality of life regarding the physiological situation (average scores, mean ± SEM, the lower the score, the better the quality of life) before and after lymphatic vessel transplantation in lymphedema of the lower extremity.

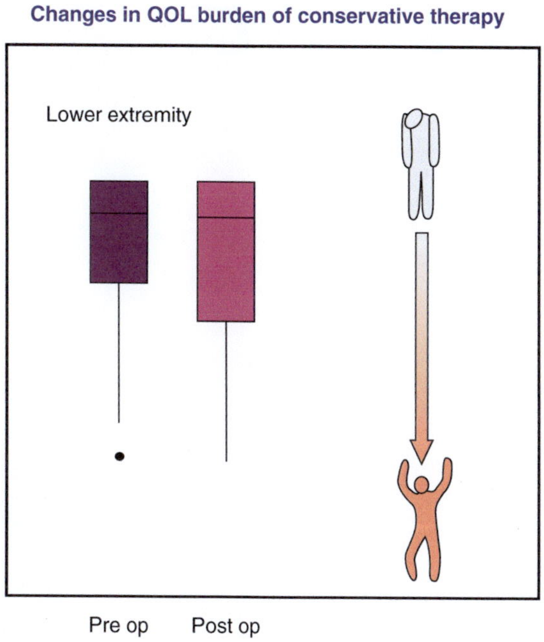

Fig. 5.22 Quality of life regarding the burden of conservative treatment (average scores, mean ± SEM, the lower the score, the better the quality of life) before and after lymphatic vessel transplantation in lymphedema of the lower extremity

He developed immediately an edema of the lower leg (Figs. 5.24 and 5.25).

5.14 Other Results

5.14.1 Treatment of Penile and Scrotal Edemas

Lymphedemas of the penis and scrotum are a challenge for conservative treatment. Manual lymph drainage and application of compression are difficult in this region. Treatment by other means is therefore of urgent need.

Lymphatic grafts are an option if the prerequisite of transposing a lymphatic vessel is given (Figs. 5.26 and 5.27).

Lymphatic vessels for transposing must be present at a neighboring thigh. Therefore, at least one leg should be free of edema, and normal lymphatic transport has to be proved by lymphoscintigraphy.

It is advisable then to use lymphatic vessels which are connected to most lateral inguinal lymph nodes. These nodes are independent from those clearing lymph out of the penile and scrotal areas. Fig. 5.28 shows the effect of short lymphatic grafts also in a long standing lymphoedema.

During surgery another prerequisite has to be given. Patent lymphatic vessels must be present at the base of the penis and detectable during surgery.

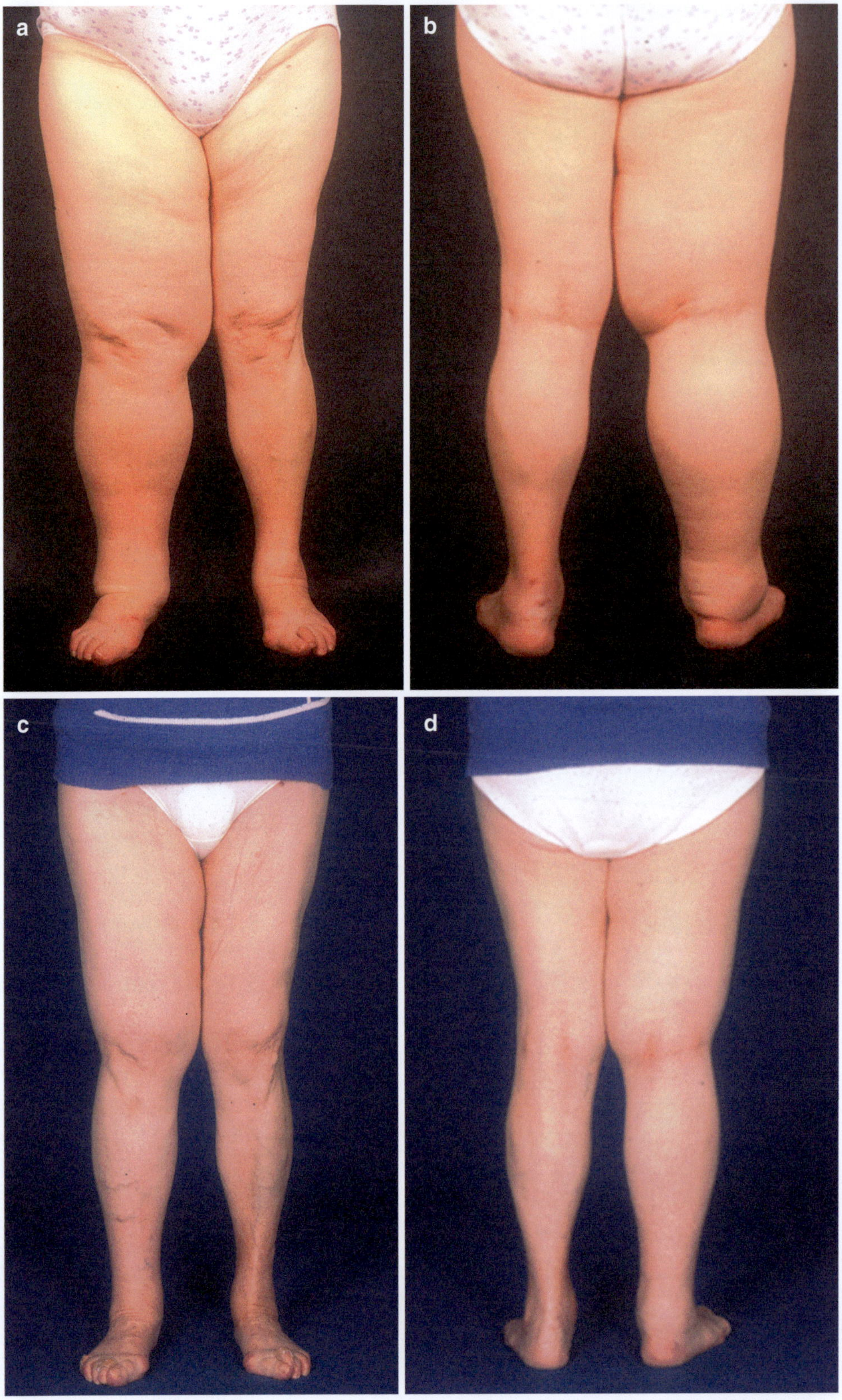

Fig. 5.23 (**a**) A 70-year-old patient with lymphedema of the right leg with after pelvic and inguinal lymph node resection. Twelve years after the onset of the edema (front view, preop). (**b**) View from behind (preop.) (**c**) 11 years after treatment by transposition of three lymphatic collectors and anastomoses to four ascending lymphatic collectors. (**d**) View from behind (postop.)

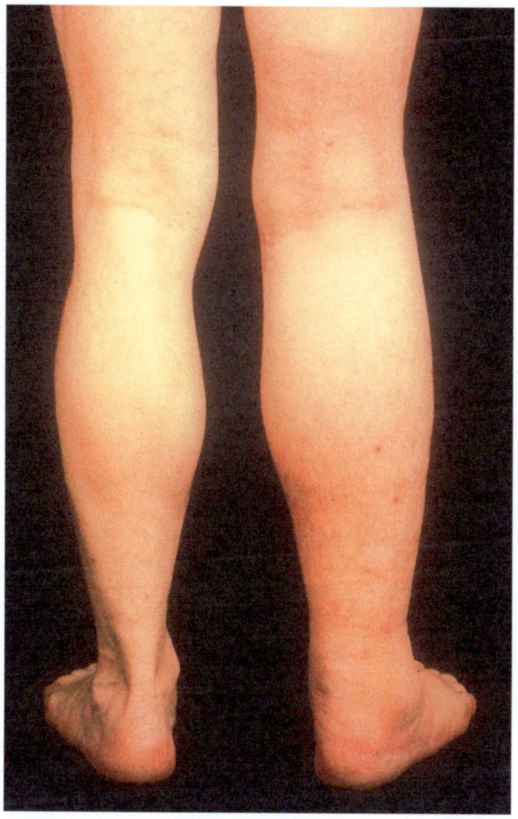

Fig. 5.24 A 45-year-old patient with edema of the right lower leg after surgical intervention at the knee

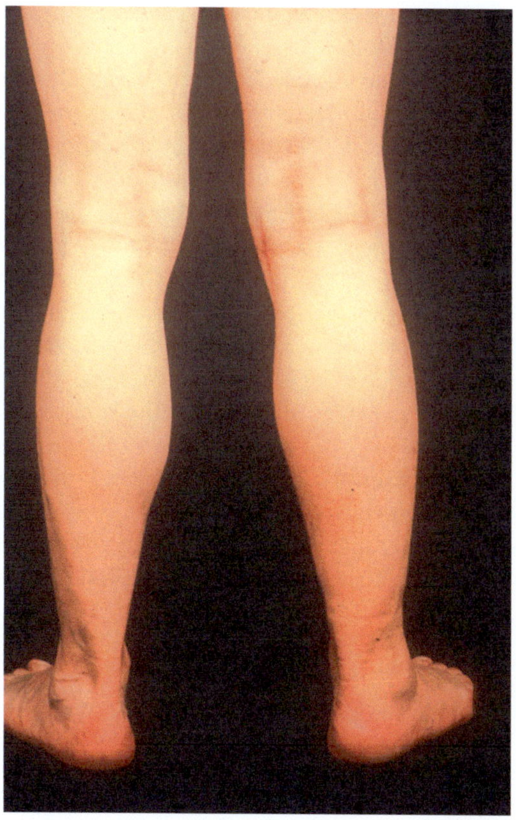

Fig. 5.25 6 months after a short lymphatic bypass by two grafts, bridging the knee area

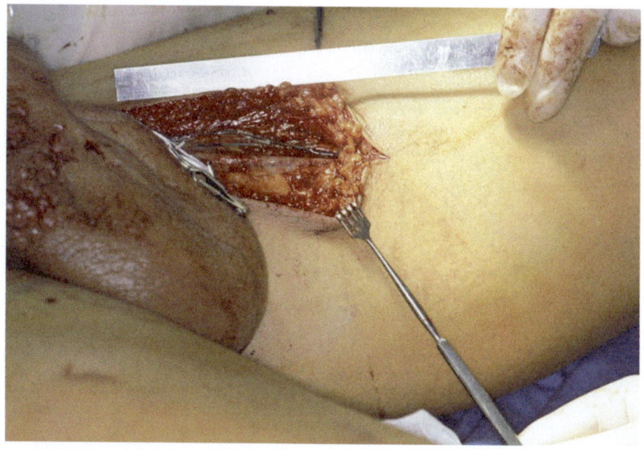

Fig. 5.26 Stained lymphatic vessels approaching the lateral inguinal lymph nodes (© Baumeister)

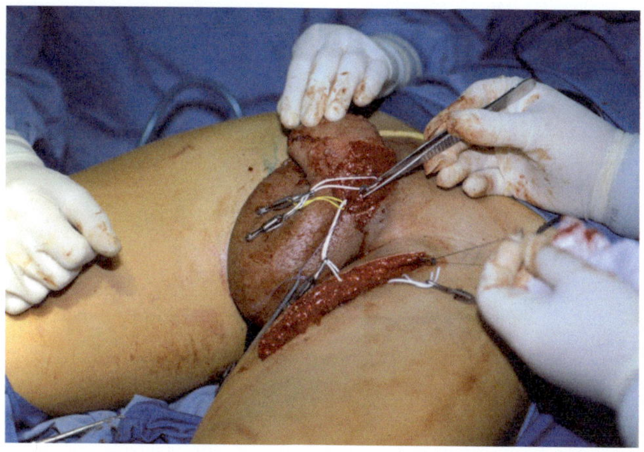

Fig. 5.27 Pulling lymphatic vessel grafts through a tube toward the anastomosing site at the base of the penis and scrotum (© Baumeister)

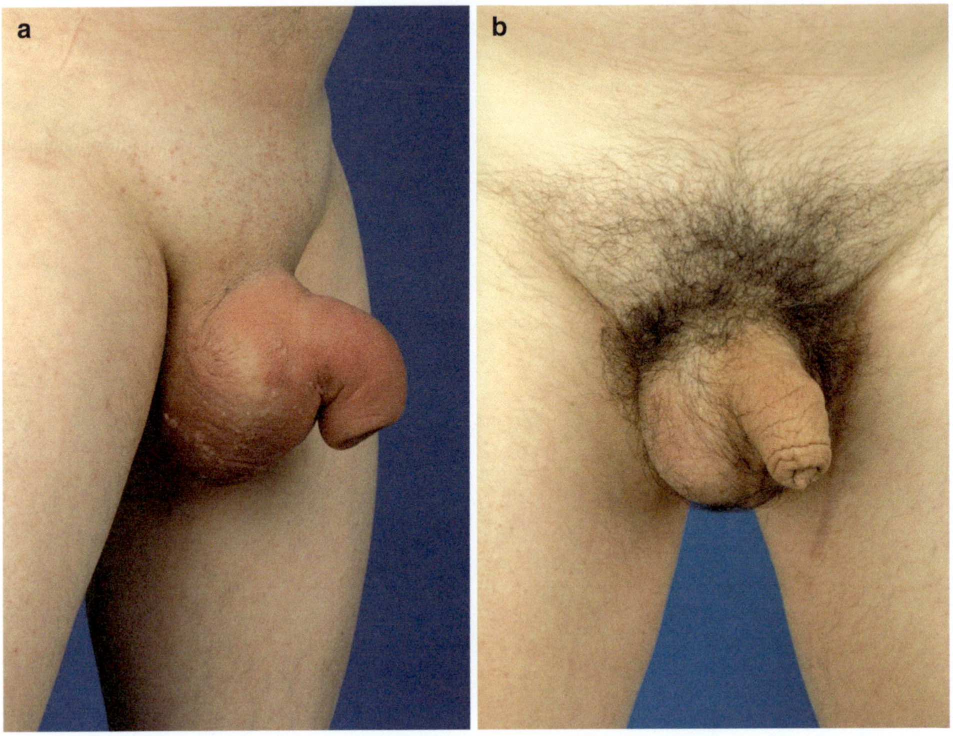

Fig. 5.28 (**a**) A 40-year-old patient, 11 years of edema of the penis and scrotum following erysipelococcus infection. (**b**) 1 year after transposition of lymphatic grafts from the left thigh (© Baumeister)

The search for lymphatic vessel is very difficult in advanced edemas. Sometimes, the tissue is so hardened that lymphatic vessels might not be found. Therefore, the option for a resection procedure should be discussed with the patient before. A scheduled combined treatment of reconstruction and resection however is not recommended.

We performed transposition of short lymphatic vessel grafts for treatment of penile and scrotal lymphedemas in ten patients with sufficient reduction of the edema in most patients.

Since volume measurements were not possible in these patients, an example may show what can be achieved by improving the lymphatic flow with the help of transposed lymphatic collectors.

The example shows a 40-year-old patient. Eleven years ago he had developed a lymphedema of the penis and scrotum after erysipelas.

5.14.2 Treatment of Lymphocele

We have treated several patients presenting with lymphocele.

According to our experience, treatment by conservative means should be considered first. Injections of high-percentage glucose (40–50 %) after emptying the lymphocele for several times are recommended.

If this does not solve the problem, microsurgical intervention should be performed.

We explored the surrounding tissue of the lymphocele after injection of dye (Patent Blue V®) in the periphery. The lymphatic vessel can be occluded and the lymphocele resected if no lymphedema is present and reconstruction is not easy.

The presence of lymphedema would indicate that lymphatic transport is insufficient. Reconstruction should be performed.

In cases of edema, the lymphatic collectors can get connected by short grafts to lymphatic vessels proximal to the lymphocele. When the lymphocele is located next to the groin and the opposite leg is without a swelling, transposing of a lymphatic collector from the healthy side would be a good solution.

If both possibilities could not be achieved, then anastomosis to adjacent veins was performed.

For these procedures MR lymphography is helpful since it can show the entrance point of single incoming collectors (Fig. 5.29).

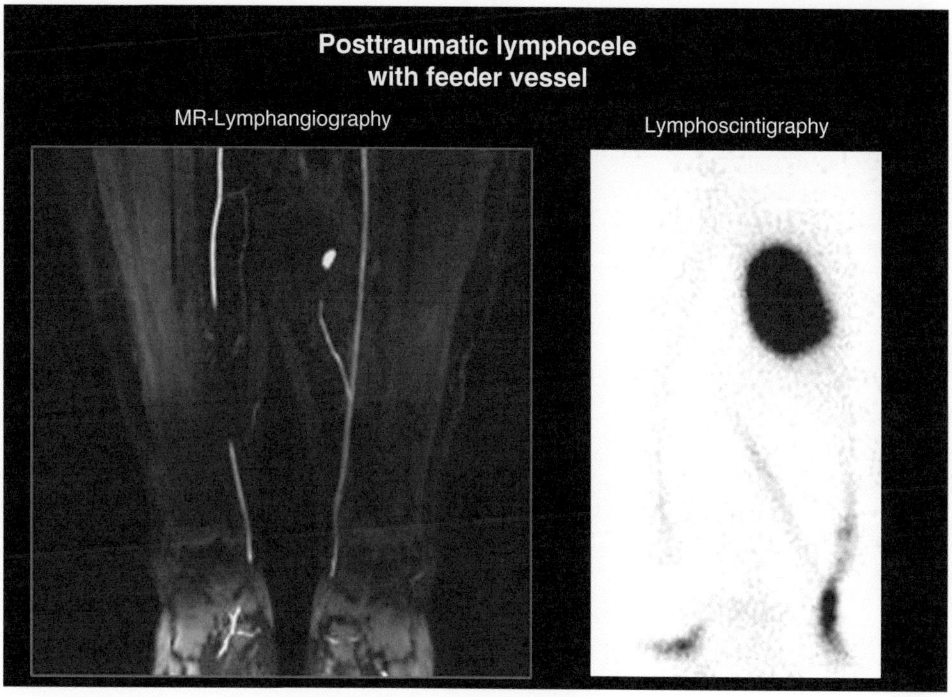

Fig. 5.29 Posttraumatic lymphocele with feeder vessel demonstrated by lymphoscintigraphy and MR lymphangiography (Courtesy PD. Dr. Notohamiprodjo)

5.14.3 Treatment of Lymphatic Fistula

Persistent lymphatic fistulas can also be treated by lymphatic microsurgery. In single patients staining of the nourishing lymphatic vessels was performed using Patent Blue V®. A superficial incision was performed around the area of the fistula. Using blunt preparation, it was searched for the stained lymphatic vessels. After having localized them, one of the procedures was chosen comparable to treatment options in lymphoceles.

In one patient with recurrent fistula at the back after axillary dissection, a lymphatic bypass procedure was asked for in a foreign hospital. The fistula subsided after bridging the axilla and finally dried up completely.

5.14.4 Complications and Their Treatments

We have noticed several complications in connection with lymphatic vessel transplantation.

In the first series of patients, we did not use antibiotics perioperatively. During that period we saw erysipelas in two patients shortly after surgery. We treated the patients with cephalosporin intravenously. After this period we gave all patients antibiotics perioperatively. From that time point, no further erysipelas in connection with the surgery was observed.

One patient developed a lymphatic cyst beneath the groin at the harvesting side. We treated the patient with repeated punctures and emptied the cyst. Thereafter the cyst disappeared without recurrence.

One patient developed signs of a venous thrombosis at the lower leg with a swelling. We treated the patient with compression garments.

One patient with an arm edema developed a hematoma above the clavicle on the night after surgery. During the intervention we found a venous bleeding which was stopped without difficulties.

References

Baumeister RGH (1981) Therapeutische Lymphgefäß-Transplantation. Fortschr Med 99:418

Baumeister RGH (1990) Die Entwicklung der autogenen Lymphgefäßtransplantation. In: Baumeister RGH (ed) Lymphologica Jahresband 1990. Medikon, Muenchen, pp 54–58

Baumeister RGH, Frick A (2003) Die mikrochirurgische Lymphgefäßtransplantation. Handchir Mikrochir Plast Chir 35:202–209

Baumeister RGH, Siuda S (1990) Treatment of lymphedema by microsurgical lymphatic grafting: what is proved? Plastic Reconstr Surg 85:64–74

Baumeister RGH, Seifert J, Hahn D (1981a) Autotransplantation of lymphatic vessels. Lancet 17:147

Baumeister RGH, Seifert J, Wiebecke B, Hahn D (1981b) Experimental basis and first application of clinical lymph vessel transplantation of secondary lymphedema. World J Surg 5:401–407

Baumeister RGH, Notohamiprodjo M, Weiss M, Wallmichrath J, Springer S, Frick A (2011) Long term results after reconstructive microsurgery using lymphatic autografts, proved by radiology and nuclear medicine. Lymphology 45(Suppl.):286–288

Kleinhans E, Baumeister RG, Hahn D, Siuda S, Büll U, Moser E (1985) Evaluation of transport kinetics in lymphoscintigraphy: follow up study in patients with transplanted lymphatic vessels. Eur J Nucl Med 10:349–352

Kuhnke E (1976) Volumenbestimmung aus Umfangsmessungen. Folia Angiol 24:228–232

Springer S, Koller R, Baumeister RGH, Frick A (2012) Changes in quality of life of patients with lymphedema after lymphatic vessel transplantation. Lymphology 44:65–71

Weiss M, Baumeister RGH, Tatsch K; Hahn K (1996) Lymphoscintigraphy for non-invasive longterm follow-up of the functional outcome in patients with autologous lymph vessel transplantation. Nucl Med 35:236–242

Weiss M, Baumeister RGH, Frick A, Wallmichrath J, Bartenstein P, Rominger A (2015) Lymphedema of the upper limb evaluation of the functional outcome by dynamic imaging of lymph kinetics after autologous lymph vessel transplantation. Clin Nucl Med 40:e117–e123

6 Reconstructive Lymph Vascular Surgery and Other Lymphedema Treatment Modalities

6.1 Resection of Accumulated Fat via Liposuction Secondary to Lymphatic Flow Reconstruction

One of the sequels of diminished lymphatic transport which causes lymphedema is the surplus of fat tissue. In advanced forms improvement of lymphatic transport alone may not be sufficient for the patient if he strives for a normal appearance of the extremity. This is highly important in particular for arm edemas since it is more difficult to hide the upper than the lower extremities.

Reducing or eliminating the surplus of fat should be done with lymphatic vessel-sparing technique, if beforehand the lymphatic transport has been restored or at least improved by lymphatic vessel grafting.

In two studies we have examined the interaction between liposuction and the main lymphatic collectors.

It was shown that, at least under tumescence conditions, the danger to harm bigger lymphatic collectors is minimal (Frick et al. 1999, 2006; Hoffmann et al. 2004).

The anastomoses are located proximal to the area of edema. Mostly they are located at the upper part of the extremity. On the other hand, liposuction is performed within the edematous region distal to the anastomosing site. Therefore liposuction without damaging lymphatic anastomoses can be applied after reconstruction.

We perform it always after a time interval. Mostly after about 1 year. The patient can experience the result of the grafting and decide if he is satisfied with it. Mostly also the effect of the grafting is documented by a lymphoscintigraphy prior to secondary liposuction.

Up to now only in one patient a lymphatic grafting was performed as secondary procedure since the liposuction was performed earlier at another institution. The first liposuction has been performed according to our proposal of a lymph-sparing liposuction.

First experiences with nine patients suffering from secondary arm edemas have been published.

The preoperative mean volume of 3273 ± 292 cm^3 was decreased to 2214 ± 149 cm^3 after reconstructive surgery followed by liposuction. This was in the range of the normal contralateral arm with 2164 ± 140 cm^3 ($P<0.001$) (Baumeister et al. 2007) (Fig. 6.1, Table 6.1).

Currently further investigations are in progress.

The example depicts the history of a 60-year-old patient suffering from a secondary lymphedema of the left arm after axillary dissection in breast carcinoma.

Figure 6.2a shows the status prior to reconstructive surgery 30 months after breast-conserving therapy which was followed by conservative treatment. The left arm is markedly swollen.

The patient underwent lymphatic grafting and 2 years later a secondary liposuction.

Figure 6.2b shows the patient in her garden in summer dress. The formerly markedly swollen left arm showed now even less volume compared to the normal arm. No additional treatment is applied.

The combination of reconstructive lymph vascular surgery and low-invasive resection of accumulated fat gives an answer to the two main problems in lymphedema, the deficiency in lymphatic transport and the accumulation of fat and fibrous tissues.

6.2 Reconstructive Lymphatic Microsurgery and Conservative Treatment

Surgical and nonsurgical treatments should not be considered contradictory to each other. They should be understood as supplementary to each other. With respect to microsurgical restoration of the lymphatic system after medical interventions, first nonsurgical treatment should be performed. During this period of about 6 months, also transient edemas may disappear and surgery can be avoided.

After reconstruction, compression garment is normally applied during a period of about 6 months in order to

R.G.H. Baumeister, *Reconstructive Lymph Vascular Surgery*, DOI 10.1007/978-3-319-31647-5_6

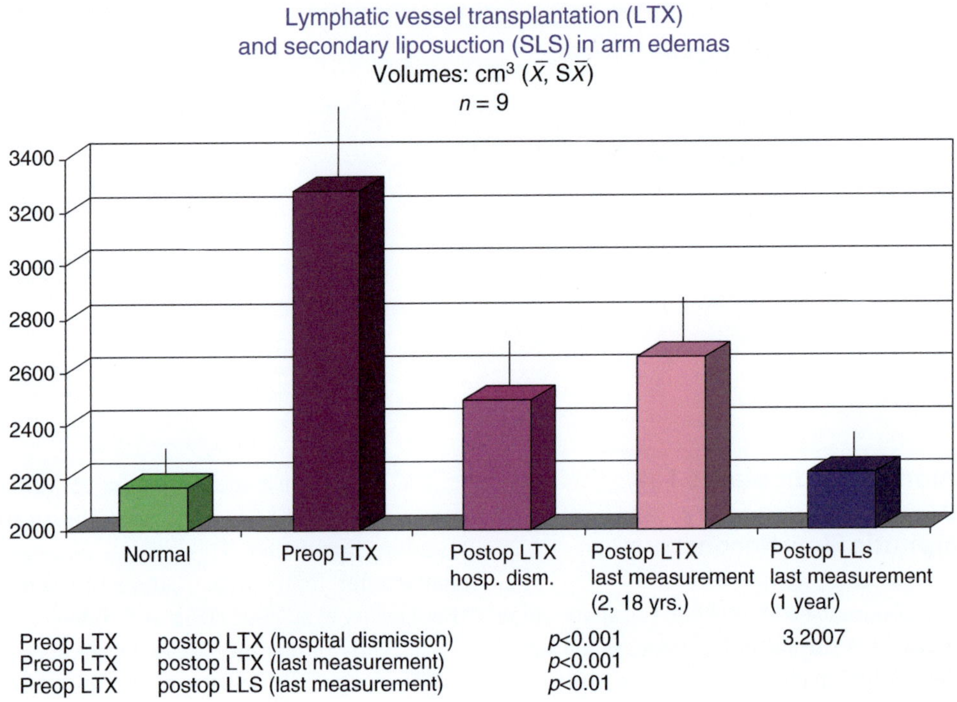

Fig. 6.1 Results of the upper limbs

Table 6.1 Mean arm volumes prior to transplantation of lymphatic vessels compared to the volume after secondary liposuction

Lymphatic vessel transplantation (LTX) and secondary liposuction (SLS) in arm edema
Volume: $cm^3 (\bar{x}, s\bar{x})$
$n = 9$

Normal	Preop LTX	Postop LTX	Postop LTX last measurement (2.18 years)	Postop LLS last measurement (1 year)
2164 ± 140	3273 ± 292	2490 ± 202	2647 ± 201	2214 ± 149
Preop LTX → postop LTX			$p < 0.001$	
Preop LTX→ postop LTX (last measurement)			$p < 0.001$	
Preop LTX→ postop LLS (last measurement)			$p < 0.001$	

facilitate the influx into the anastomoses by increasing the pressure within the tissue distal to the anastomoses.

During these six postoperative months, we do not recommend manual lymph drainage. The net effect of the reconstructive procedure can be observed without interference with another lymphatic transport-stimulating technique.

Additionally, we had not seen a difference between two groups: with and without additional manual lymph drainage in a pilot study with 20 patients.

After this postoperative period of about 6 months, the transient compression garment is removed, and possible worsening is carefully watched.

Thereafter about one-third of the patients experience stable conditions and do not need any further additional treatment. One-third use additional compression especially under working condition, and one-third need compression therapy and manual lymph drainage as well.

Already in an early study on 34 patients with arm edemas, we saw similar courses. All patients had compression therapy and manual lymph drainage prior to surgery. After the period of 6 months with the routine compression, 14 patients could leave out completely the compression. Nine used it only temporarily during strong working conditions. Eleven patients used it furthermore continuously.

Twenty-four out of the 34 patients were able to omit the manual lymph drainage after the reconstruction completely. Ten patients restarted the additional treatment by manual lymph drainage (Baumeister 1990).

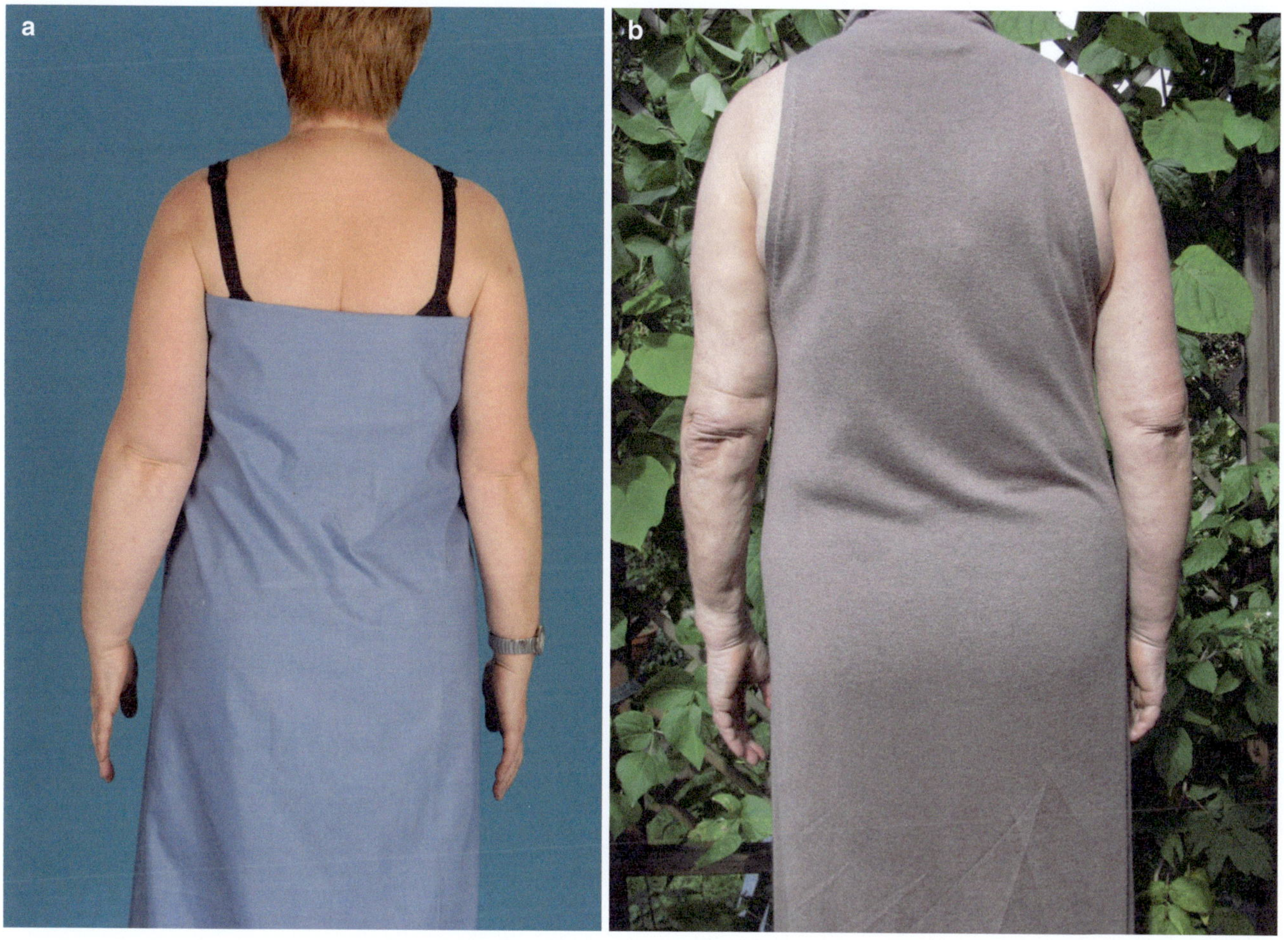

Fig. 6.2 (**a**) A 60-year-old patient with lymphedema of the left arm after breast-conserving therapy. (**b**) 5 years after secondary liposuction following lymph vascular reconstruction without additional treatment (© Baumeister)

References

Baumeister RGH (1990) Physikalische Therapie und Mikrochirurgie des Lymphödems- Gegensatz oder Ergänzung. In: Baumeister RGH (eds) Lymphologica Jahresband 1990. Medikon, Muenchen

Baumeister RGH, Wallmichrath J, Weiss M, Frick A (2007) Reconstructive microsurgery and treatment of secondary tissue changes in lymphoedema. Lymphology 40 (Suppl):541–543

Frick A, Hoffmann JN, Baumeister RGH, Putz R (1999) Liposuction Technique and Lymphatic Lesions in Lower Legs- An Anatomical Study to Reduce its Risks. Plast Reconstr Surg 103:1868- (k)

Frick A, Baumeister RGH, Hoffmann JN (2006) Liposuction technique and lymphatics. In: Shiffmann MA, Guiseppe D (eds) Liposuction principles and practice. Springer, Berlin/Heidelberg, pp 26–29

Hoffmann JN, Baumeister RGH, Fertmann J, Putz R, Frick A (2004) Tumescent and dry liposuction of lower extremities: differences in lymph vessel injury. Plast Reconstr Surg 113:718–724

MIX
Papier aus verantwortungsvollen Quellen
Paper from responsible sources
FSC® C105338

If you have any concerns about our products,
you can contact us on
ProductSafety@springernature.com

In case Publisher is established outside the EU,
the EU authorized representative is:
Springer Nature Customer Service Center GmbH
Europaplatz 3, 69115 Heidelberg, Germany

Printed by Libri Plureos GmbH
in Hamburg, Germany